The Interval Training Workout

Joseph T. Nitti, M.D., is uniquely qualified to write about interval training (I.T.), being a physician who has studied many aspects of human physiology over the past 20 years. As a national class-distance runner, he utilized I.T. for over a decade to become a qualifier for the 1992 Men's U.S. Olympic Trials at the marathon distance. His initial interest in exercise training led to a bachelor of science degree in kinesiology with a specialization in exercise physiology from UCLA. Dr. Nitti currently manages patients' pathophysiology of disease as a board-certified cardiovascular anesthesiologist in private practice. He lives in southern California with his wife, Kimberlie Nitti, an avid amateur athlete and personal trainer who specializes in wellness programs for women.

The authors wish to dedicate this book to our role models, the elite athletes
and coaches who have, through critical thinking and years of work, pushed the
envelope of human endeavor. These individuals have inspired us to push our own
limits and allowed us to learn more about ourselves than we ever thought possible.

Ordering

Trade bookstores in the U.S. and Canada, please contact:

Publishers Group West
1700 Fourth Street, Berkeley CA 94710
Phone: (800) 788-3123   Fax: (800) 351-5073

Hunter House books are available at bulk discounts for textbook course adoptions; to qualifying
community, health care, and government organizations; and for special promotions and fund-
raising. For details please contact:

Special Sales Department
Hunter House Inc., PO Box 2914, Alameda CA 94501-0914
Phone: (510) 865-5282   Fax: (510) 865-4295
E-mail: ordering@hunterhouse.com

Individuals can order our books from most bookstores or by calling toll-free:

(800) 266-5592

THE
INTERVAL TRAINING
WORKOUT

Build Muscle and Burn Fat
with Anaerobic Exercise

Joseph T. Nitti, M.D.

and

Kimberlie Nitti

Hunter House PUBLISHERS

Hunter House Inc., Publishers
PO Box 2914
Alameda CA 94501-0914

Library of Congress Cataloging-in-Publication Data

Nitti, Joseph T.
   The interval training workout : build muscle and burn fat with anaerobic exercise / Joseph T. Nitti and Kimberlie Nitti.
      p. cm.
   Includes bibliographical references.
   ISBN-13: 978-0-89793-328-5 (cl) — ISBN-13: 978-0-89793-329-2 (sp) —
   ISBN-13: 978-0-89793-327-8 (pb)
   ISBN-10: 0-89793-328-1 (cl) — ISBN-10: 0-89793-329-X (sp) — ISBN-10: 0-89793-327-3 (pb)
   1. Exercise. 2. Aerobic exercises. 3. Cardiovascular fitness. I. Nitti, Kimberlie. II. Title.
RA781.15 .N55 2001
613.7'1—dc21   2001016621

Project Credits

Cover Design: Peri Poloni, Knockout Design
Book Design and Production: Jinni Fontana
Photographs: Anne Marie Fox
Developmental Editor: Jeff Campbell
Copy Editor: Bevin McLaughlin
Proofreader: John David Marion
Acquisitions Editor: Jeanne Brondino
Associate Editor: Alexandra Mummery
Editorial and Production Assistant: Emily Tryer
Acquisitions and Publicity Assistant: Lori Covington
Marketing Assistant: Earlita Chenault
Customer Service Manager: Christina Sverdrup
Order Fulfillment: Joel Irons
Computer Support: Peter Eichelberger
Administrator: Theresa Nelson
Publisher: Kiran S. Rana

Manufactured in the United States of America

9 8 7 6 5 4 3 2   First Edition   08 09 10 11 12

Contents

Acknowledgments

We wish to thank the many friends and family members who generously played a part in making this book possible. Most of all, we are grateful to all our models, whom we shamelessly strong-armed into service: Mark Luevano, Annetta Luevano, Dr. Gary Nitti, Wendi Nitti, and Vic Simonian. Thanks also to Joe Douglas of the Santa Monica Track Club, Carl Lewis, Jenny Spangler, Anne Marie Fox, Mattias Persson, Michael Gunn, Melanie Winstead, and Chuck Crossland of 24-Hour Fitness/Santa Monica.

Important Note

The material in this book is intended to provide a review of information regarding fitness training. Every effort has been made to provide accurate and dependable information, and the contents of this book have been compiled through professional research and in consultation with medical professionals. However, always consult your doctor or physical therapy practitioner before undertaking a new exercise regimen or doing any of the exercises—or following the suggestions—contained in this book.

The authors, publisher, editors, and professionals quoted in the book cannot be held responsible for any error, omission, or dated material in the book. The author and publisher are not liable for any damage or injury or other adverse outcome of applying the information in this book in an exercise program carried out independently or under the care of a licensed trainer or practitioner. If you have questions concerning the application of the information described in this book, consult a qualified and trained professional.

As a world-class athlete and Olympic champion, I've found that people around the world are curious to peek inside the head of an elite athlete and find an answer to one particular question: what's the secret?

The truth is, there isn't one.

I didn't win those medals because I trained at altitude, or had to run back and forth to school as a child, or took any performance-enhancing drugs or supplements. There are only three things that make a great athlete: good genes, a strong work ethic, and an intelligent, well-crafted training program.

It's been said, "To become an Olympic athlete, choose your parents well." There may come a day when genetic engineering is perfected, but for now we all have to work with what we're born with. What you *can* control is how hard you are willing to work for your physical goals.

It isn't easy, pushing your body to higher heights, faster times, greater distances. There have been many, many days when I felt too tired or too sore to work out or just plain didn't feel like doing it. But I did it anyway. That's what you do if you want to win gold at the Games or attain a personal best in a sport or just make your body fitter and stronger than ever before. Working hard and, even more importantly, working *smart*—this is truly the stuff of champions.

Not everyone can be an elite athlete. But knowing how to train like one, that's a whole different story. *The Interval Training Workout* is the next best thing to having your very own coach. The techniques found in this book aren't new or revolutionary, as interval training has been used for decades by the world's greatest athletes. What is special about this book is that it presents interval training as a complete program for athletes of *all* abilities. *The Interval Training Workout* can teach you how to train like a world-class athlete—the rest is up to you. If you can dream great dreams and have the dedication, courage, and determination to make them come true, you can be one of the few to reach your full physical potential. Who knows how far you'll go? Set your goals high—then go out and attain them. That's what being an athlete is all about.

Carl Lewis has won more Olympic gold medals than any American in history. He has been ranked number one in the world in the 100 meters, 200 meters, and long jump multiple times. He is considered by many to be one of the greatest athletes of all time.

It's not the years, it's the mileage.

—Indiana Jones

Despite the overwhelming hype and promise of the fitness boom, most people never meet their fitness and weight loss goals. The complaints are all too common: "I run 15 miles a week but I haven't lost any more weight." Or, "How can I still be out of shape when I work out on the stair climber 30 minutes every day?"

Why is this?

It's because most people do no more than mildly exert themselves at the same comfortable, steady pace each time they work out. It may work for a while, but as millions of frustrated exercisers have discovered, it doesn't work for long. The unfortunate thing is that most people have never been taught how to improve.

What is clearly needed is an exercise routine that:

- Is scientifically and clinically proven to build muscle, burn fat, and improve the body's cardiovascular system

- Can be adapted for use with different aerobic activities, such as running, walking, cycling, or swimming or for workouts using fixed exercise machines (such as stair climbers, stationary bicycles, treadmills, cross-country ski machines, or elliptical trainers)

- Doesn't require any special or expensive equipment

- Can be done alone or with others

- Is designed so you can progress at your own pace

- Can be used by anyone in reasonable health with a basic foundation of fitness

- Offers a variety of workouts to keep things interesting

- Provides a clear measure of physical improvement

- Gives maximum results in minimal time

These very elements form the basis of the I.T. Program, a practical, easy-to-understand, scientifically and clinically proven fitness plan based on the training methods used by the fittest, leanest people on earth: elite athletes.

I.T. stands for "interval training," a technique originally developed in the 1930s. Until then, athletic training for endurance events was a bit haphazard, and many athletes who found their way to the top of the awards podium were victorious simply because they had the good fortune to have superior genetics. You either had it from birth or you didn't—the ability to go faster wasn't considered attainable by any other means.

Fortunately, two German track coaches dared to think differently. As exercise physiologists, they had a theory that if a runner practiced doing brief segments of his regular workouts at a faster "race pace," he could later string together all those fast segments in actual competition to achieve a better overall time.

It worked. Varying the degree of effort used within a single workout (fast "repetitions" followed by slower recovery "intervals") produced spectacular results. World records began to improve dramatically and athletes all over the world scrambled to adopt the revolutionary interval training method for themselves. One such individual was British medical student Roger Bannister. In 1954, after using the principles of I.T. in his daily one-hour training regimen, he went on to run the world's first sub–4-minute mile. This set an exciting new benchmark for athletic achievement—and human potential.

Today, every top endurance runner, cyclist, and swimmer aiming for peak performance uses some form of interval training. That's a good enough recommendation for us. But what if you're not an elite athlete? No problem. The same physiologic principles apply to almost everyone, from weekend warriors to national-class marathoners. It's not necessary to be in stellar shape to benefit from interval training. Just the opposite, in fact: the I.T. Program is designed to help you attain superior fitness.

Until now, there's never been a single, authoritative source that presented the basic training principles of elite athletes in a way that could be adapted by others interested in better health and fitness. But after Joseph qualified for the '92 Olympic Trials, so many people began to ask for advice about their own training that we started writing down our notes—and the I.T. Program slowly began to take shape. Those who were motivated enough to follow the program described in this book went on to achieve—and sometimes even surpass—their health and fitness goals. We were motivated to publish the I.T. Program because it worked for them, and we're confident it can work for you, too.

—Joseph and Kimberlie Nitti

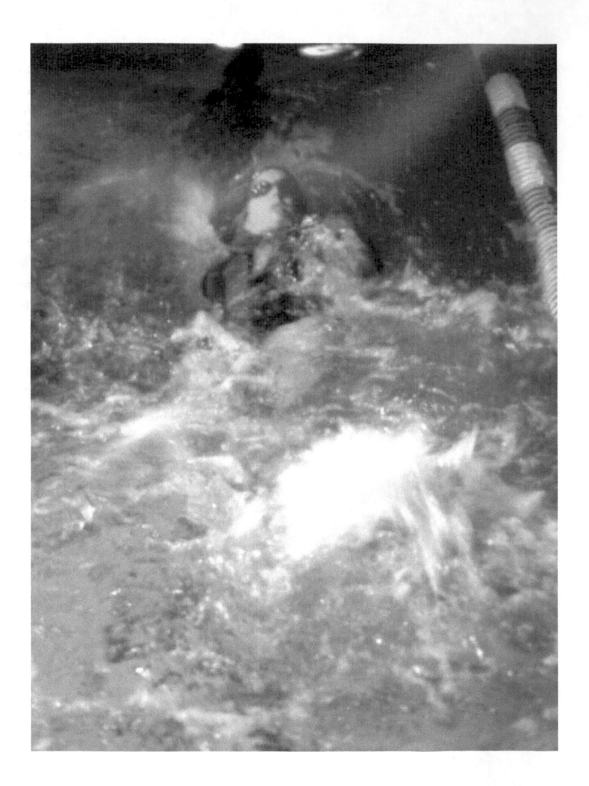

1

I.T. Basics: The Science Behind the Fitness

Over the years, various fitness "gurus" have had a major influence on the American public. Charles Atlas, Jane Fonda, Richard Simmons, and Billy Blanks, among others, offered a fitness program designed to improve health, build muscle, and burn calories. Each one of these exercise entrepreneurs became a household name to millions of faithful fans. But, oddly enough, the person who probably had the most influence on fitness in this country might very well be someone you've never even heard of.

Dr. Kenneth Cooper launched one of the biggest fitness revolutions in history with his book *Aerobics,* published in the late 1960s. Cooper's book popularized the notion that moderate aerobic exercise (strictly defined as exercise done "with oxygen") performed three to four times a week for 20 minutes was all it took to improve health and fitness. Aerobics became hugely popular and inspired the jogging craze of the 1970s and the "power walking" fad that followed. People were understandably enthused about an exercise plan that required little more than lacing up a pair of sneakers, wasn't too physically taxing, didn't take all day, and even packed a bit of an endorphin kick. It sounded like the discovery of the Holy Grail of physical fitness, and, to some degree, it was. Aerobic devotees enjoy fairly decent returns for their rather minimal efforts, becoming fitter, managing their weight better, and enjoying healthier lives.

In fact, aerobics has become such a part of the cultural lexicon that today the very word calls to mind images of spandex-clad bodies sweating to the beat of loud music in packed exercise studios. But the aerobics movement also includes the many dedicated fitness buffs who run, walk, cycle, swim, and use fixed exercise machines. This massive group of well-intentioned, health-oriented individuals probably includes you, the reader of this book.

So the question is, with all this exercising going on...

Why aren't there more people out there in better shape?

Two words:

Plateau effect.

The Plateau Effect

The "plateau effect" is a rather disheartening leveling off of fitness as measured by such things as exercise tolerance, weight control, and athletic performance. Anyone who works out consistently has probably experienced this dreaded plateau to some degree. You're exercising as much as ever, but instead of improving, you're unable to budge those last few pounds or advance to a tougher level of step class or swim a mile any faster than you could swim it months ago.

Why is this?

It's because your exercise program is too limited.

The bottom line is that purely aerobic exercise can only take the body so far, even if you had a whole day, every day, to devote to working out. Relying solely on moderately paced, moderately difficult exercise, as most people do, will never, ever give you anything more substantial than (yawn) moderate results. You'll definitely be in better shape than a beer-swilling, channel-surfing couch potato—of course—but you won't ever be considered very fit. Unfortunately, most people have never been taught to exercise any other way.

Does aerobic exercise work? Sure.

But interval training works better.

Interval training (I.T.) makes the most of the limited amount of time most of us have available for exercise. Instead of squandering this time on comfort zone exercise, the I.T. Program devotes a couple sessions a week to more challenging workouts. These workouts use brief bursts of higher-intensity activity to generate powerful physiologic processes, which result in decreased body fat and increased fitness and strength. I.T. helps you work smarter with what time you have and ultimately rewards you with better results.

Why I.T. Is Superior to Purely Aerobic Exercise

There is no question that interval training is superior to purely aerobic exercise. This has been proven both in the stadium and in the laboratory. Basically, I.T. delivers remarkable results by using the body's natural ability to adapt to physical stress. The I.T. Program is based primarily on several scientifically proven mechanisms.

I.T. Increases Human Growth Hormone

One way the body deals with the stress of higher intensity exercise is by secreting hormones, such as Human Growth Hormone (HGH). This naturally occurring anabolic (or "building") hormone stimulates muscle growth by encouraging the creation of protein. HGH also makes fats more available as fuel for the body by increasing

their presence in the bloodstream. Simply put, HGH builds muscle and burns fat, which is exactly what most people are looking to get out of their workout program. Several experts have even touted HGH as the secret to slowing the aging process and enjoying a longer, fuller life. It's not too surprising that some Olympic-caliber athletes have been banned for cheating with illegal injections of HGH.

Fortunately, you can steer clear of needles and get the same performance-enhancing benefits by doing interval training, which increases HGH. Blood levels of HGH have been shown to rise significantly during and immediately after interval training. This is substantially different from purely aerobic exercise, in which HGH levels remain the same both during and after a workout. No matter what level of fitness you're at or what type of exercise you do, I.T. boosts HGH production like no other legal substance. I.T. also releases other useful hormones such as corticotropin, cortisol, and catecholamines, all of which help to mobilize fats as a source of energy.

I.T. Burns Calories

I.T. burns calories because it gets you exercising at higher intensities for brief chunks of time. This extra effort takes more energy than the plodding pace of aerobic exercise because it taps larger, less efficient muscle fibers that aren't frequently used. And, using more energy means you're burning more calories.

Even better news: I.T. revs up your metabolism. After intense exercise, the body needs extra calories as it works to repair muscles, replenish energy stores, and restore the body to its normal state again. Since this can take from several hours to a full day, you'll keep on burning calories long after the workout is over. That doesn't happen with purely aerobic exercise. Over the course of the I.T. Program, resting metabolism increases along with lean muscle mass, because muscle needs additional calories to fuel its everyday metabolic functions. All this calorie burning and muscle building ultimately results in a leaner, fitter body. You can't beat that.

The Power "A"s: ATP, Aerobic, and Anaerobic

The words "cellular metabolism" may trigger haunting memories of high school biology class, with all those charts of Kreb's Cycles and other scary stuff that you promptly forgot after final exams. For anyone serious about athletics, however, a simple explanation of how the power "A"s generate energy within exercising muscles might be interesting.

For starters, you need to know that ATP stands for "adenosine triphosphate," and an ATP molecule is the basic unit of cellular energy. Say you're walking down a street. In order to move, ATP needs to be broken down in the muscles to provide the required energy. But there are only a few seconds worth of ATP available in your cells, so more has to be made, pronto—otherwise you'll stop moving. The primary energy provider, aerobic metabolism, kicks in. "Aerobic" means "with oxygen," and aerobic metabolism combines oxygen with carbohydrates, fats, and proteins to create ATP. Aerobic metabolism is pretty darn efficient, in that it can produce a whopping 38 ATP by combining a single molecule of glucose (a form of carbohydrate) with oxygen. Since there's an abundance of oxygen available when you're walking at an easy pace, you can keep creating enough ATP to plod along for quite some time.

Now say you start jogging. The faster pace requires more energy, which means there's

(continued on facing page)

I.T. Taps Larger Muscle Fibers

Interval training requires both small and large muscle fibers. Smaller muscle fibers are better at utilizing oxygen and are employed mostly for aerobic exercise, while larger fibers generate more power and are used mainly for more strenuous anaerobic (meaning "without oxygen") exercise. Since the larger fibers cannot use oxygen efficiently, they tend to fatigue quickly—which explains why you can only sprint so far, so fast, before you're exhausted and gasping desperately for air. Doing only moderate aerobic workouts all the time means that larger muscle fibers are more or less ignored, and they'll eventually shrink and weaken from lack of exercise. Use it or lose it, in other words. Interval training, on the other hand, uses small and large muscle fibers. Making use of these

(continued from facing page)

less oxygen available for use. You start breathing harder, trying to get more oxygen into your lungs, and your heart rate speeds up to deliver that oxygen to working muscle cells. The oxygen then moves to the cell "powerhouses" (mitochondria), to crank out enough ATP to meet the muscles' energy needs. This is considered an aerobic workout, exercise that is done at an intensity that can be adequately fueled with oxygen.

Pick up the pace to a sprint. Now you are generating maximum ATP using oxygen (i.e., aerobically), but it just isn't enough to maintain the higher speed. Here's where the anaerobic system kicks in. Anaerobic metabolism converts carbohydrates and some fats into ATP without using any oxygen whatsoever and provides enough energy to keep you sprinting for a short time. But there's a cost. For one thing, the anaerobic system is extremely inefficient—it can only generate a measly two (two!) ATP from a molecule of glucose. It also produces lactic acid, a nasty substance that causes your legs to burn after a short burst of sprinting. Eventually, the acidity shuts down muscle cell activity, causing your muscles to fail and forcing you to slow down. This allows the lactic acid to disperse and recovery to occur as oxygen levels catch up again to meet the body's energy needs. For all its limitations, the anaerobic system is the primary way to create energy in larger muscle fibers during very high-intensity activity, such as interval training.

larger fibers makes them more efficient and results in stronger muscles that are better able to handle heavy-duty exercise.

I.T. Means Greater Fitness in Less Time

There's no question that aerobic exercise done regularly improves the body's cardiovascular system. But sooner or later there comes the dreaded fitness plateau, when improvement seems to grind to a halt. The I.T. Program is scientifically proven to break through this sort of barrier and provide you with greater fitness in less time. Studies of aerobically trained runners show that after a few months of interval training they are able to pump more blood and deliver more oxygen to their muscles, generating more energy than ever before. The I.T. Program also incorporates extra-long sessions of aerobic exercise—known as "XL Workouts"—which help the body generate energy in other ways. Here's how: during aerobic exercise, oxygen travels from the lungs via the blood to working muscles, where it's passed along from blood capillaries to muscle mitochondria (cell "powerhouses" that use oxygen to convert food into energy). XL Workouts help beef up capillary density and the number and size of mitochondria, so more oxygen can be used by the muscles, which results in more efficient energy production. Basically, having more energy to power a workout results in greater fitness for you, because you can exercise at higher intensities for longer periods of time.

With all this going for the I.T. Program, why wait? If you're anything like most people, you're looking for results, yesterday. Let's get started!

Your Notes:

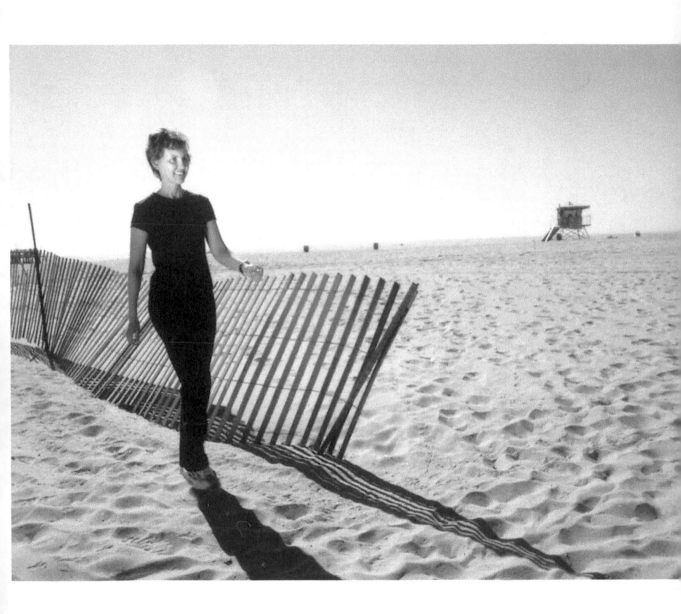

2

Before You Start:
Building the Foundation

The I.T. Program can benefit almost any healthy person, from beginning exercisers to world-class endurance athletes. In fact, most athletes you see participating in the Olympics or other major events use some form of interval training in their own workout programs. That's not bad company to be in.

But even these paragons of fitness didn't start off doing I.T. from Day 1. They first had to develop a foundation of aerobic fitness that allowed them to physically and psychologically manage the higher intensity levels that interval training demands.

A consistent program of aerobic exercise, even at a low level of effort, results in several encouraging changes:

- a more efficient heart and circulatory system
- improved oxygen delivery and utilization by the muscles
- stronger muscles, tendons, ligaments, and bones

- improved body composition (less fat and more muscle)

- better self-image and overall sense of well-being

Doing nothing but aerobic exercise may be enough for people who aren't out to become superfit. But for more motivated exercisers, aerobic training is mainly a springboard to the I.T. Program and its proven formula to control weight and attain maximum fitness.

Before starting the I.T. Program, you must be able to complete 30 minutes of continuous exercise at least three times a week for 4 consecutive weeks.

This continuous exercise can be any aerobic activity (such as walking, running, cycling, or using a stair climber) done at any intensity level, provided it lasts for 30 minutes. Already at this level of conditioning? You're probably ready to start doing I.T. If you don't have the recommended foundation yet, follow the Aerobic Base Program described later in this chapter. You'll be ready to step up to the I.T. Program in just 8 weeks. In either case, read the medical precautions section below before moving on to your first workout session.

Medical Precautions

From blisters to stress fractures to heart attacks, there's always a possibility of some pain or injury with physical exertion. It may be necessary to get a green light from your doctor to ensure your body is up to the rigors of a new, strenuous exercise program. The American College of Sports Medicine (ACSM) has two useful pre-exercise evaluations we've adapted here. They can help determine if you might be at risk for coronary artery disease or a disease of the cardiovascular and pulmonary systems.

Don't be overly concerned if you do need to see a doctor—a thorough medical history and physical exam may be all that's needed to get a thumbs-up to work out. Some simple blood tests or an electrocardiogram or a chest X ray may also be required, just to rule out the possibility of major organ disease (affecting such things as your heart, lungs, liver, kidneys, endocrine system, or blood). Even if you feel perfectly healthy, you might need to do an exercise stress test if your doctor feels you may be at risk for myocardial ischemia (lack of oxygen to the heart) or heart failure (inability of the heart to manage exercise stress). A stress test simply involves walking or jogging on a treadmill while your

Coronary Artery Disease Risk Factors

Family history: Myocardial infarction [heart attack], coronary revascularization [heart by-pass surgery], or sudden death [due to cardiac arrest] before 55 years of age in father, brother, or son, or before 65 years of age in mother, sister, or daughter

Cigarette smoking: Current cigarette smoker or those who quit within the previous 6 months

High blood pressure: Systolic blood pressure [upper number] of greater than or equal to 140 mm Hg; or diastolic [lower number] blood pressure of greater than or equal to 90 mm Hg, confirmed by measurements on at least two separate occasions; or taking anti-hypertensive [high blood pressure] medication

High cholesterol: Total serum cholesterol of greater than 200 mg; or high-density lipoprotein cholesterol [HDL, or "good" cholesterol] of less than 35 mg; or on lipid-lowering medication. If low-density lipoprotein cholesterol [LDL, or "bad" cholesterol] measurement is available, use more than 130 mg as measure rather than total cholesterol of more than 200 mg

Impaired fasting glucose: Fasting blood glucose [test taken after 6 hours without food] of greater than or equal to 110 mg confirmed by measurements on at least two separate occasions

Obesity: Body Mass Index of greater than or equal to 30 kg/m squared [measured by taking your weight in kilograms and dividing it by your height in meters] or waist girth of more than approximately 40 inches

Sedentary lifestyle: Persons not participating in a regular exercise program or meeting the minimal physical activity recommendations from the U.S. Surgeon General's report (30 minutes or more of moderate physical activity on most days of the week)

*Reprinted with permission from JAMA and Lippincott Williams and Wilkins (*ACSM's Guidelines for Exercise Testing and Prescription, Sixth Edition,* American College of Sports Medicine, Lippincott Williams and Wilkins, Baltimore, Maryland, 2000)

Major Signs or Symptoms Suggestive of Cardiovascular and Pulmonary Disease

- Pain or discomfort in the chest, neck, jaw, arms, or other areas that may be angina ["heart pain" due to lack of oxygen]
- Shortness of breath at rest or with mild exertion
- Dizziness or syncope [fainting]
- Ankle edema [swelling]
- Palpitations or tachycardia [rapid heart rate]

- Orthopnea [shortness of breath when lying flat] or paroxysmal nocturnal dyspnea [awakening at night short of breath]
- Intermittent claudication [pain in a limb with use, such as leg pain when walking]
- Known heart murmur
- Unusual fatigue or shortness of breath with usual activities

Consult your doctor before starting any new exercise program if you:

- Have any risk factors or symptoms listed above
- Have diabetes or any known cardiovascular (heart), pulmonary (lung),

hepatic (liver), renal (kidney), or thyroid disease

- Are 70 years or older (your doctor may want to do a physical exam and perhaps some lab tests to rule out any disease that might be present but not causing symptoms)

Other age considerations:

If you are 45–70 years old and male, or 55–70 and female, without any of the listed risk factors or medical limitations, go ahead with low to moderate aerobic activity (defined by the ACSM as any comfortable level of intensity that can be sustained for up to 60 minutes, starting slowly and progressing gradually).

If you are 45 years or older and male, or 55 or older and female, or if you have two or more coronary artery disease risk factors, consult your doctor before doing any exercise vigorous enough to tire you after 20 minutes. Your age group is more at risk for underlying heart

disease, so be sure to have a physical exam and an exercise stress test before starting the I.T. Program.

If you are younger than 45 years and male, or younger than 55 and female, with no more than one risk factor, move ahead with low to moderate aerobic exercise such as that found in the Aerobic Base Program, outlined in this chapter. If you already have a solid aerobic foundation, you're ready to start the I.T. Program.

*Reprinted and adapted with permission from JAMA and Lippincott Williams and Wilkins (*ACSM's Guidelines for Exercise Testing and Prescription, Sixth Edition,* American College of Sports Medicine, Lippincott Williams and Wilkins, Baltimore, Maryland, 2000) heart is monitored for changes. The test may also include an echocardiogram to look for cardiac abnormalities such as decreased function and heart valve disease. It's a painless procedure done with a special probe (it looks like a small pressing iron) that's placed on your chest to generate an ultrasound image of the heart. Your doctor can interpret the results and help construct an exercise program you can feel confident and comfortable doing.

Aerobic Base Program

Don't worry if you suspect you aren't quite ready for interval training. If you don't have any medical limitations, the simple, 8-week Aerobic Base Program will get you on the road to better health and fitness. This program, like the I.T. Program, is based on "progressive overload," in which muscles are challenged with a gradually increasing level of effort over time. You start off easy and do a little more each week, factoring in some rest and recovery between steps, until you achieve your goal: 30 minutes of continuous aerobic activity, 3 to 4 times a week. Once you can do that, you're ready to move on to the full-fledged I.T. Program.

Here's how to get started.

First, choose a form of exercise. What interests you? What's most convenient? How available is equipment or a gym? If you like exercising outside, consider walking, jogging, swimming in a lake or outdoor pool, or cycling on an open road or trail. If you prefer an indoor environment or a more social setting, try a well-equipped gym with treadmills, stair climbers, exercise bikes, cross-country ski machines, or elliptical trainers. Some people use their local shopping mall as a warm, dry, safe place for a good brisk walk. If it works for you, why not? The idea is to choose an activity you can do consistently 3 to 4 days a week.

Start off doing just a single exercise, such as walking or cycling or stair climbing (later, when you start doing the I.T. Program, you may want to cross train by adding a few more activities). At this point, the level of intensity is not that important because your goal is merely a consistent 30-minute workout. (Once you can do that 3 to 4 times a week, and you don't have any medical limitations, you're ready to move on to the I.T. Program.) For now, just concentrate on completing the exercise at a pace that is comfortable—and enjoyable—for you.

Week 1

Day 1: 10 minutes continuous activity

Day 2: Rest day

Day 3: 10 minutes continuous activity

Day 4: Rest day

Day 5: 15 minutes continuous activity

Day 6: Rest day

Day 7: Rest day

Week 2

Day 1: 15 minutes continuous activity

Day 2: Rest day

Day 3: 15 minutes continuous activity

Day 4: Rest day

Day 5: 20 minutes continuous activity

Day 6: Rest day

Day 7: Rest day

Week 3

Day 1: 20 minutes continuous activity

Day 2: Rest day

Day 3: 20 minutes continuous activity

Day 4: Rest day

Day 5: 25 minutes continuous activity

Day 6: Rest day

Day 7: Rest day

Week 4

Day 1: 25 minutes continuous activity

Day 2: Rest day

Day 3: 25 minutes continuous activity

Day 4: Rest day

Day 5: 30 minutes continuous activity

Day 6: Rest day

Day 7: Rest day

Weeks 5 through 8

Day 1: 30 minutes continuous activity

Day 2: Rest day

Day 3: 30 minutes continuous activity

Day 4: Rest day

Day 5: 30 minutes continuous activity

Day 6: Rest day, or 15–30 minutes of continuous activity

Day 7: Rest day

There are a few things to keep in mind as you undertake this Aerobic Base Program.

If at any time you experience pain in your chest, jaw, upper back, or left arm, or a severe, sudden shortness of breath, stop immediately and call for medical assistance. These may be signs of myocardial ischemia (decreased oxygen supply to your heart).

If you are physically unable to complete a workout anytime during the first 4 weeks, decrease the effort level of the next workout or move back 1 week in the sequence.

Have fun! The time you spend doing this comfortably paced exercise can be used constructively to consider new ideas, come up with solutions for problems at home or at work, listen to favorite music, or even read magazines. Use it to clear your head or hang out with friends—taking a walk together instead of chatting over cups of coffee helps keep things interesting and gives an added boost of motivation, too.

Practical Advice: Shoes and Athletic Apparel

When it comes to exercise, having the right shoes and athletic apparel can make all the difference between a comfortable, enjoyable workout and one that's miserable because of blisters, chafing, or dampness.

Choose Comfort over Style

Always opt for comfort over style. There's no need to spend a fortune on designer stuff with logos all over the place.

Wear Layers

Being nice and toasty at the beginning of a workout means you're overdressed. You'll be hot and sweaty in no time, and later wet, cold, and maybe dehydrated, too. This is why marathoners compete in 40-degree weather in nothing more than shorts and singlets. Wear layers so you can ditch them as things heat up.

Choose Materials that "Breathe"

Clothing should allow heat and sweat to evaporate, wicking moisture away from the skin. Look for synthetics specially designed for this purpose, or a synthetic/cotton blend. Clothing that is made of 100 percent cotton is fine for easy workouts in which you don't sweat much, or for top layers that can be shed. Otherwise, avoid having it next to the skin, as it soaks water up like a sponge.

Don't Experiment on Hard Workout Days

Avoid experimenting with new shoes and new clothes on hard workout days. Wear stuff that's well broken in, especially if you're competing in a race.

Buy Well-Built, Supportive Shoes

A pair of well-built, supportive running shoes is great for running, walking, group aerobics classes, and using fixed exercise machines. Plan to do several different activities? A cross-training shoe might be an even better option. Be prepared to spend at least $50—anything less tends to be poorly constructed or lack decent support. It's a good investment and may save you a heap of pain and doctor bills.

Buy Shoes from Specialty Stores

Stores that specialize in running shoes offer the best selection and consultants to guide you through the mind-boggling assortment of options out there. Take the shoes for a test jog right there in the store; a good store will encourage this sort of thing. If the shoes slide or pinch or feel weird on a little test jog, they'll make you truly miserable after 30 minutes of exercise!

Stick with the Shoes You Like

Once you find a brand and style of shoe you like, stick with it. Save money on future shoes by ordering through wholesale catalogs, such as Road Runner Sports. And, be sure to replace shoes often enough—

when the rubber treads on the soles start to look worn and smooth or the fabric uppers start ripping, it's time for a fresh pair.

Practical Advice: Where and When to Work Out

Your options for where and when to work out may be limited, depending on the exercise you do. Swimmers need a lap pool or open water; cyclists need long, traffic-free stretches of road; users of fixed exercise equipment usually need to belong to a health club or gym.

Location, Location, Location

Walkers and runners have the most flexibility when it comes to locations to work out. All they need are a road or trail or track and a good pair of shoes. For those doing the Aerobic Base Program (and for all beginning exercisers), the ideal training surface is smooth and flat. More advanced walkers, runners, and cyclists can incorporate more varied terrain into their workouts, such as hills, steep grades, or rough mountain trails. I.T. Workouts can be done anywhere, but a measured area is best, such as a track or a footpath with mile markers. Experiment with new places on easy workout days but stick with the tried and true for more challenging workouts. Psychologically, it's easier to work hard in a familiar environment, where you know things like exactly how far there is to go and how long it takes to get to the next turn. On days when the weather is lousy or it's too inconvenient to drive to your favorite workout spot, exercising indoors on a treadmill or other machine may be your best bet.

Working Out Indoors

If you plan to work out indoors with a stair climber, stationary bike, treadmill, or elliptical trainer, you'll most likely have to work out at a gym. Even if you're considering buying a piece of equipment for use at home, it's a good idea to test drive it for a few weeks at a gym before forking over a hefty wad of cash. Some tips for finding a good gym to join:

Is it close to home or work?

Does it have lots of aerobic exercise machines? Are they usually occupied at the time of day you want to use them?

Is there a time limit on machine use? Many gyms have a 20- or 30-minute limit on machines during peak hours. You'll eventually get on, but you may have to interrupt a longer workout session until another machine becomes available.

Is there good air circulation? Some gyms keep the aerobic area as warm as the weight lifting area. This isn't a good idea, as it can lead to overheating.

Are the contract terms favorable? Do you have to lock-in to a long-term commitment? Can you use the membership at other clubs?

Can you get a free pass to try out the place for a few days before signing on the dotted line?

What's involved in getting out of the contract? You might decide later to join a different gym or take up an outdoor activity instead.

Crunched for Time

Who isn't crunched for time? Unless you have Olympic aspirations or a generous trust fund, it won't always be easy to find time to squeeze in a workout. But with a little sacrifice and creativity, it's entirely possible to find 30 to 60 minutes 4 to 6 days a week to improve your fitness, if you really want to.

Exercising consistently requires a good dose of realism. Are you a morning person or a night person? When do you have the most energy, and the least? Can you find an hour before work? On your lunch break? After class? Figure out a schedule you can stick to and don't procrastinate when exercise time rolls around—the longer you stall, the harder it is to get out the door. Sometimes just putting your shoes or swimsuit on is the hardest thing about working out—once you make that mental commitment, it's simply a matter of following through. Or, at least that's what we keep telling ourselves. For some strange reason, it usually works.

No matter how committed you are, though, there are days you just can't work out. You might be sick or traveling or tied up with a huge project at work. Other times your body and mind may sort of shut down and force you to take a day off, despite all your best intentions. Let it happen and don't cave into guilt or try to overcompensate at your next workout. If you find yourself skipping more and more workouts for no apparent reason, you might be pushing too hard physically or have a problem with motivation. Step back, re-evaluate what you're doing, and move on from there.

Special Considerations for Women

Personal Safety

For personal safety, stay aware of your surroundings whenever exercising outdoors. Leave the headphones at home so you can hear if someone is behind you, and try not to be out alone after dark or in remote or deserted areas. Stick to well-lighted, familiar routes and do whatever you can to avoid looking vulnerable, lost, or anxious.

Fertility Problems

Some female athletes are concerned that intense exercise will cause fertility problems. Interval training can cause some women to have more menstrual irregularities or temporary disruptions in their periods. Some of these disruptions include the rather well-publicized amenorrhea (no period), as well as a shortened luteal phase and reduced ovulation, any of which can make getting pregnant more difficult. In simple terms, the added physical stress that a rigorous workout places on the body causes it to shift into an energy-saving mode. This diverts energy from reproductive functions so it's available for exercise instead. The result? A skipped menstrual cycle here or there or the absence of a period altogether.

If you're trying to get pregnant, don't worry. In most cases, all that's needed to get a regular cycle going again is to ease up on your training—it's not necessary to stop completely—and make sure you're eating enough. Try backing off on at least one of your more intense workouts each week and eat an extra snack or two, about 300 to 400 calories worth. Chronically missed periods can cause bone mass to decline and lead to stress fractures and osteoporosis, so see your doctor to rule out other problems and to get your periods back on schedule again.

Exercising while Pregnant

If you don't have any high-risk conditions and it's okay with your doctor, you don't have to give up exercise while pregnant. On the contrary, studies show that exercising while pregnant has many benefits: active women seem to have calmer babies, fewer complications, shorter labor and deliveries, and are less likely to develop gestational diabetes or other problems. It helps get your pre-baby body back more quickly after delivery, too, and that's certainly a plus. But save the intense training of the I.T. Program for after the baby arrives. Pregnancy puts enough stress on the body as it is, and topping it off with a demanding exercise program may be harmful to the developing baby. Stick to moderate exercise only during pregnancy and avoid fatigue, heat, and dehydration. Be sure to consult your doctor immediately if you ex-

perience any faintness, pain, absence of fetal movement, or sudden swelling, or a racing heart during or after a workout. It may be nothing, but it's best to play it safe for the full 9 months.

Special Considerations for Teenagers

Diet

It takes a lot of energy to be a teenager and even more to be a teenage athlete. Diet is especially important for teens, as they need more calories and nutrients than people at any other stage of life. The average 11- to 14-year-old boy needs at least 2,500 calories a day, and boys 15 and older need about 2,800. Add 1,000 calories or so on top of that for those playing sports or training with the I.T. Program. Girls need at least 2,200 calories a day, plus an additional 800 if they are doing a lot of exercise. That's a serious amount of food, and any parent of a teenage athlete probably has the grocery bills to prove it.

The majority of these calories shouldn't come from junk food. Teenagers should take healthy snacks to school to have throughout the day and should eat a variety of foods. Dairy products are good sources of calcium, which is especially important for teenagers who are still growing bone. Of course, every high school student we know would much rather chug a soda than a carton of milk, but building up bone mass during adolescence can help prevent exercise-related problems later on in life. So keep nagging.

I.T. and the Teenage Athlete

With some common sense, the I.T. Program can be used safely and to great effect by teenagers, and many high school swimming and running programs already use similar training techniques. Adolescents do need to be especially cautious of overuse injuries, poor coaching, improper technique, pushing beyond simple fatigue, and participating in unhealthy forms of competition. If you are a concerned parent or guardian, here are some points to consider if your teen is in an athletic training program:

- Teenagers are not small adults. Some aches and pains are expected for every athlete, but a teenager's complaints should be given extra-careful consideration. Undiagnosed, untreated injuries can cause permanent damage to developing bones, muscles, tendons, and ligaments and can impede proper growth. Never allow a teen to work "through the pain."

- Encourage flexibility and strength training so teens can better maintain muscle balance and suppleness. The joggers you see today who can barely touch their shins (much less their toes) began losing this ability in high school. Start good habits early to avoid overuse injuries later on in life.

- Young athletes of the same age can differ greatly in size and physical maturity and may try to perform at levels they're not ready for.

- Teens are more likely than adults to become overheated and develop heat-related illness. Vigorous activity on very hot days should be limited to early morning or late afternoon (preferably after sunset) when temperatures are cooler, and teenage athletes should be encouraged to drink lots of fluids.

- Teenage athletes need proper guidance and training, and that means qualified coaching. Oftentimes schools and sports clubs make their own hiring decisions and parents have little say in the matter. But talk to other parents and observe a few workouts to see if the coach teaches proper technique and keeps workouts to a reasonable level of difficulty. A good coach tailors workouts to each athlete's ability and knows when enough is enough. Joseph Nitti's high school track workouts and overall mileage increased yearly in a structured fashion that kept him healthy, adequately rested, motivated, and competing successfully.

- Teenagers should be allowed to explore a variety of athletic activities. Whatever sport they choose, foster an atmosphere of healthy competition that stresses self-reliance, confidence, cooperation, and positive self-image over winning at all costs.

Considerations for Older Exercisers

Most active people intend to continue exercising for the rest of their lives. And these days it's truly possible—people are living longer, healthier lives, practicing good preventative care, benefiting from the advances of modern medicine, and working out at ages thought unimaginable years ago. The I.T. Program is not designed for the frail elderly, but for healthy individuals,

it can have a positive impact on many common geriatric problems: it can reduce and prevent muscle weakness, decreased muscle mass, low bone density, cardiovascular deconditioning, and poor balance. If you play it smart and maximize what you have, there's no reason why you shouldn't be able to keep on using the I.T. Program far past your retirement party. Here are some specific considerations for older exercisers to keep in mind:

- Aerobic capacity declines after the ripe old age of 30, but it's possible to slow the slide. An active middle-aged person can be more physically fit than a college-aged sofa surfer, so it's worth-while to make exercise a lifelong habit. Anaerobic capacity declines at an even faster rate, but that's usually because people do less high-intensity exercise as they age. Keeping up your I.T. Workouts will hold losses to a minimum.

- The older you get, the longer it takes to recover from workouts. You can't really overcome this, unfortunately— you just have to learn to accommodate it. After a tough workout or a race, give yourself enough time to fully rest before the next hard effort. You may need to incorporate more Active Rest Days into your I.T. Program.

- Joints get stiffer and muscles becomes less flexible with time, so buckle down and start stretching on a regular basis.

- It's easier to gain fat and lose muscle mass with age. Metabolism slows by about 5 percent every 10 years, and strength, speed, and stamina start to dwindle along with bone tissue. It's just a part of life, but you can do a lot to stave off these changes by adding strength training to your exercise program.

- For active people, particularly competitive athletes, it can be hard to keep up motivation as the years go by. Priorities change, you can't train as hard, and you have more injuries or nagging aches and pains. But try to remember that a good exercise program keeps you healthier and active far longer than hanging out in a front porch rocking chair ever will. Some older athletes actually get a kick out of competing in higher age brackets, because they come away with more trophies and fanfare than they ever managed in their salad days. A good attitude and a sense of humor are key if you want to keep making the most out of your body and your life.

Older people do have more sports-related injuries, many stemming from years of athletic wear and tear and age-related changes that make tissues more prone to injury. But that's no reason to stop exercising; just take a few extra precautions:

- Follow the medical precaution guidelines outlined earlier in this chapter.

- Make sure your program includes cardiovascular work, strength training, and flexibility exercises.

- Pay attention to symptoms. If you ever have pain in your chest, left arm, jaw, or upper back, or severe shortness of breath or faintness, see your doctor immediately.

- Pay attention to pain, especially if it's in your joints. See a doctor right away if the pain is only on one side or doesn't go away after a day or 2. Also, take more Active Rest Days and allow yourself at least 1 full day off each week.

Your Notes:

_____

_____

_____

_____

_____

_____

_____

_____

_____

_____

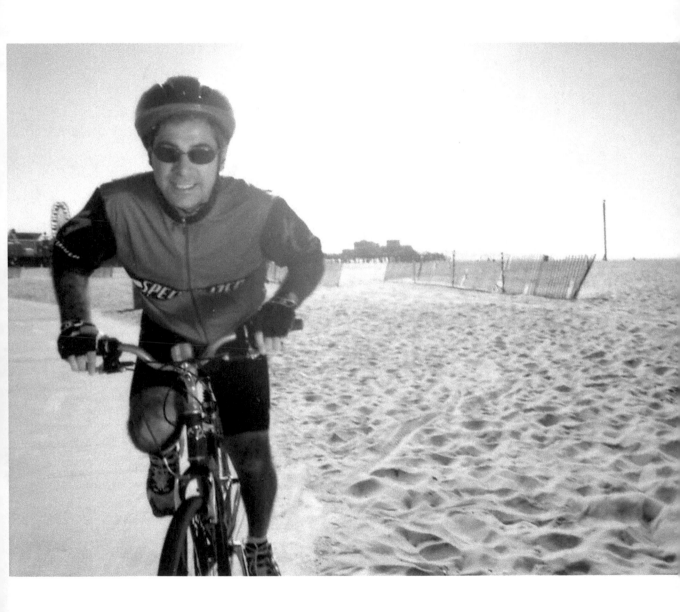

3

Your First I.T. Workout

Interval training is a whole different animal from purely aerobic exercise. In fact, an alternate title for this book could very well be *Anaerobics,* as the goal of an I.T. Workout is to fatigue the body with brief periods of higher-intensity effort. This greater level of effort triggers biochemical, cardiovascular, and muscular changes to create a fitter, leaner body. The result: maximum gain, the most efficient way possible.

A firm grasp of the building blocks that form the I.T. Workout will help you get the most out of training. Some terms used throughout this book are explained below.

Repetition (or Rep)

A repetition is the high-intensity portion of an I.T. Workout, a period of greater exertion lasting from 30 seconds to about 5 minutes. Depending on how challenging you want your workout to be and how much time you have, you do a certain number of repetitions with a lower-intensity rest interval between each one. For example, a runner might run 8 fast repetitions of 400 meters (1 lap around a regulation-size track), with intervals of 200 meters (a half lap) of slow jogging in between each rep.

A repetition is measured by distance or by time. Any predetermined distance, such as 400 meters, can be used. This method obviously works best in a measured setting where exact distances can be easily monitored, such as a high school track, a standard size swimming pool, or a stationary bicycle or treadmill with an electronic mileage function.

Measuring a repetition by time is just as effective and is more flexible in terms of where it can be done. For instance, a cyclist might do 5 repetitions in a high gear, each lasting 2 minutes, with 3-minute intervals in a much lower gear to recover between reps. Use a stopwatch when it's hard to judge exact distances, such as on a footpath without clear mile measurements or when using a stair climber.

Keeping track of the number of repetitions you manage to complete during each I.T. Workout is an easy way to chart progress and see how much your conditioning is improving.

Interval (or Rest)

An interval is the recovery period between the more strenuous repetitions and is also measured by distance or by time. It's called "interval training" and not "repetition training" for good reason: the interval determines how much rest the body gets between repetitions, and that greatly influences the intensity of each rep. For instance, if the interval between 1-minute runs is 10 minutes long, there's ample time to rest and prepare to run the next rep very fast. But if there's only 30 seconds to rest, running that next rep at the same fast pace is a much bigger challenge. Intervals are usually done as "active rest," such as slow walking or jogging; this actually speeds the clearance of lactic acid better than resting at a complete standstill does. A possible exception to this is swimming in a pool in which lanes are assigned according to speed. In this case, the interval may be a rest at the nearest wall so as not to hinder other swimmers.

Intensity

Intensity is the degree of effort used to complete a repetition and can be determined several ways.

Time—Covering a certain distance in a specific amount of time, such as swimming 50 meters in 1 minute.

Level—Graduated steps of effort electronically programmed into certain fixed exercise machines. For example, doing a 2-minute repetition on a stair climber at level 8, followed by a 2-minute interval at an easier, lower level.

Pulse—Heart rate during or immediately after completing a repetition. Accurate readings during exercise require a heart rate monitor, which for most people is an unnecessary expense (see pages 31 and 32).

Subjective assessment (or "feel")—This rather hard-to-define gauge of intensity is commonly used by advanced-level athletes. With some experience, it can be a very useful method.

How do all these elements—repetitions, intervals, intensity—come together? Some practical examples might help. Here's how an I.T. Workout for a stair climber might look jotted down on paper:

5 x 1 minute at level 8/2 minutes at level 4

Translation? The first half refers to the repetition: 5 high-intensity 1-minute reps on level 8. The other half refers to the interval: 2 minutes of active rest done at the easier level 4 between the repetitions.

Here's an example using distance instead of time. A world-class distance runner who wants to run 6 1-mile repetitions at a 4½ minutes per mile pace might have a workout that looks like this:

6 x 1 mile in 4:30/440-yard jog

By manipulating repetition length, repetition number, level of intensity, and interval length, you can easily design I.T. Workouts using combinations as infinite as the imagination. Dial things up or down depending on your level of conditioning, how strong or tired you feel, how much time you have to exercise, and so forth.

Ready to give I.T. a try?

With interval training, it's always better to take a few minutes to think through the workout before starting. Here's how to go about it, step by step.

Determine Total I.T. Time or Distance

To figure out how much of a workout should actually be devoted to I.T., just take your total workout time, subtract the time needed for warm-up and cooldown, and use the remaining time for I.T. For instance, for someone who usually exercises on a stair climber for 30 minutes at level 3, an I.T. Workout might be broken down like this:

10-minute warm-up

15 minutes of interval training (repetitions followed by intervals)

5-minute cooldown

Total: 30 minutes

For a swimmer who swims 40 laps daily, a first I.T. Workout might be:

10-lap warm-up

24 laps of I.T.

5-lap cooldown

Total: 39 laps

Warm-Up and Cooldown

It's a good idea to adequately warm up and cool down whenever doing interval training. Because I.T. Workouts are done at a higher intensity, it's important for muscles to be warm and supple before starting. A brief warm-up kicks fuel stores into gear, lessens the chance of injury, and maximizes the quality of the workout. Elite athletes sometimes spend up to 45 minutes warming up before a challenging session, but 5 to 15 minutes of activity at a slow pace is fine for most people. For example, a runner planning a 3-mile or 30-minute I.T. Workout might warm up with a 1-mile (10-minute) jog. Afterward, a slow 5- to 10-minute cooldown lets the body gradually return to its pre-exercise state, helping speed recovery between workouts.

Choose Either Time or Distance

If you exercise in a measured setting, such as a track or a lap pool or on a bike with an odometer function, it's easy to use specific distances. Otherwise, you'll want to go by time, which can be used in any environment.

One-Minute Reps, 2-Minute Intervals

There are good reasons for starting off with 1-minute repetitions and 2-minute intervals, and they will be discussed in more detail later. For now, keep it simple and fit as many sets of 1-minute repetitions and 2-minute intervals as you can into the workout time you have. For the stair climber example above, the I.T. portion of the workout is broken down like this:

10-minute warm-up at low intensity

5 repetitions of 1 minute at a higher level, with 2-minute intervals at a lower level between reps

5-minute cooldown at low intensity

Total: 30 minutes

The same ratio works for distance-based workouts, too, although there's a bit more estimating that needs to be done. For instance, if it normally takes 75 seconds to run a ½ lap around a track at your baseline aerobic exercise pace, do a half lap for your repetition distance as well (since you'll run it at a faster pace, it will take closer to 60 seconds to complete the same distance). The same thing goes for estimating interval distances. If it usually takes 90 seconds to swim 1 lap at your baseline aerobic exercise pace, use 1 lap as the distance for your I.T. intervals (intervals are done at an even slower pace, so the 1 lap will take closer to 2 minutes to complete). Rounding off a bit is perfectly okay.

A swimmer who normally swims 90-second laps will have a first I.T. Workout that looks like this:

10-lap warm-up at a slow pace

12 repetitions of one lap at a higher intensity, with slower 1-lap intervals between reps (this assumes that you can swim both fast and slow in a given lane; otherwise, spend 2 minutes at the wall between reps)

5-lap cooldown at a slow pace

Total: 39 laps

Step Up/Step Down to Determine Intensity

Figuring out just how hard to push yourself is one of the more challenging aspects of the I.T. Program, so the best strategy is to keep things simple. Intensity can be measured numerous ways, but when you're just starting out, it's a good idea to go with the step up/step down method.

Step up/step down is just what it says: after warming up, step up the intensity one notch from your baseline aerobic workout pace for repetitions, and step down one level from baseline pace for the intervals. Here are a few examples to better illustrate how it works:

Walking

Briefly warm up at an easy walking pace, then jog the repetitions (a step up in intensity) and walk slowly for the intervals (a step down in intensity).

Running

Warm up with a slow run, then stride out—a fast pace, but not as fast as full-out sprinting—during the rep (a step up in intensity) and jog the intervals (a step down in intensity).

Swimming

Warm up by swimming several easy laps, then increase the stroke rate so each repetition is about 10 to 30 percent faster than your baseline aerobic exercise pace (a step up in intensity). For the intervals, decrease the stroke rate to 20 to 40 percent below your baseline aerobic pace (a step down in intensity).

Cycling

Warm up with some easy spinning in your usual gear, then shift 2 to 3 gears higher for the reps. Shift down 2 or 3 gears below your baseline gear for the intervals.*

Fixed Exercise Machines

Warm up at a low level of resistance, then, for the repetitions, increase the effort level so it's about 20 to 40 percent harder than your baseline aerobic exercise pace (a step up in intensity). For instance, if you normally cruise at level 4, do the reps at level 5 or 6. For the intervals, decrease the effort level about 20 to 50 percent below your baseline aerobic pace (a step down in intensity). Again, if your usual level is 4, try level 2 or 3 for the interval.*

*Note: Be sure to keep the turnover (the number and depth of steps for stair climbers, rpms for bikes, strokes per minute

What Does an I.T. Workout Feel Like?

Unlike the steady pace of an aerobic workout, in which you feel pretty comfortable throughout, an Interval Training Workout entails a seesaw of fatigue and recovery that may be a tad hard to get used to at first. That first hard repetition is likely to be much more difficult than you imagined. Don't worry—your larger muscle fibers are just protesting as they shift into full work mode, and things generally smooth out by the 2nd and 3rd repetitions. Your mission is to maintain the same level of intensity for each rep you do, which isn't as easy as it sounds.

As an I.T. Workout progresses, the repetitions will feel like they're getting harder and the intervals will feel shorter and shorter. Just remember that the benefit of this workout comes when you are tired, not when it's easy! Strangely enough, you may experience a sort of second wind towards the end of your workout and feel an urge to increase the intensity of the repetitions. Try to avoid doing this and focus instead on finishing feeling strong. You can always make adjustments to your next workout.

for rowing machines) at the same level as in your baseline aerobic workout. Otherwise, it's easy to cheat by going slower.

Remember, these are just guidelines. Precise intensity levels aren't of such great importance for your first I.T. Workout. Instead, focus on getting used to alternating levels of hard and easy exercise.

Once You Finish

Most people come to the same conclusion after they finish their first I.T. Workout:

It's tiring!

I.T. is definitely more physically challenging than the moderate aerobic exercise that most people do for each and every workout session. Any physical activity is better than nothing, of course, but for those who are dedicated to achieving greater fitness in less time, a leisurely stroll with a book on a treadmill just isn't going to cut it.

Why You Don't Need a Heart Rate Monitor

With the I.T. Program, you don't need to invest in an expensive heart rate monitor (or do complicated mathematical formulas to figure out target training zones or anything like that). The manufacturers tout these monitors as crucial pieces of equipment,

First I.T. Workout Checklist

- **Warm-up:** Do at least 5 minutes (preferably 10) at a slightly lower intensity than your baseline aerobic exercise pace

- **Repetition:** Go 1 minute (or equivalent distance) at a step up from baseline aerobic exercise pace

- **Interval:** Go 2 minutes (or equivalent distance) at a step down from baseline aerobic exercise pace

- **Repeat:** 1 1-minute repetition/2-minute interval cycle as many times as the I.T. portion of your workout allows (I.T. portion = your baseline aerobic exercise workout time, minus warm-up and cooldown time)

- **Cooldown:** Continue exercising for at least 5 minutes at a very low intensity level

particularly for beginning exercisers, who tend to overdo things in the first few weeks. But different people have different heart rate tolerances during workouts. For instance, a world-class runner can sustain 80 to 90 percent of his maximum heart rate for the 2-hours-plus it takes to finish a marathon. A novice runner can handle such a high rate for only a few minutes. So which runner should be training at 80 percent of his maximum heart rate? The heart might pump oxygenated blood like crazy, but that doesn't mean the muscles can use that oxygen effectively. Heart rate also fluctuates with temperature, stress, dehydration, and lack of sleep, so it's a complicated indicator. If you aren't sure how to interpret it, a heart rate monitor won't do you much good.

Is it possible for an inexperienced exerciser, or any nonelite athlete, to intuitively work out at an appropriate intensity without a heart rate monitor? Certainly. The I.T. Program helps you gain more experience listening to your own body, so you'll know how it feels to be exercising at an optimal training rate. Of course, if you need to be extra cautious due to health problems (if you have heart disease, for example, or high blood pressure), a heart rate monitor might very well be a useful tool to have on hand. Check it out with your doctor.

Your Notes:

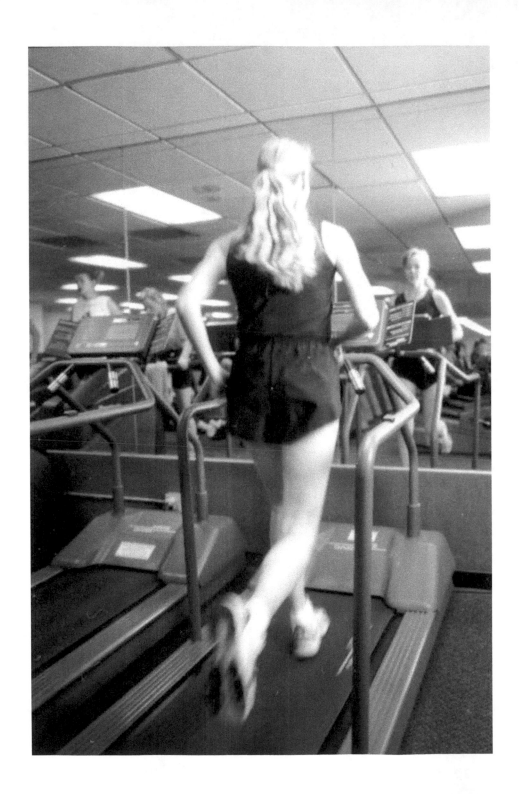

4

Customizing Your I.T. Workout

The beauty of the I.T. Program is in being able to adjust any of the four variables—number of repetitions, length of repetitions, interval length, and intensity—for a full range of training options, from easy to ultra-demanding.

Of course, this flexibility can also be a curse. Having too many choices leaves some people with option paralysis, like kids in a candy shop flummoxed by a huge display of lollipops. But knowing how and when to change each variable of the I.T. Program is crucial to making headway towards your fitness goals. Develop a starting point—an optimal I.T. Workout—then experiment a bit, customizing your workout one adjustment at a time. Your I.T. Workout is a work in progress, slowly evolving as your fitness improves.

Developing an Optimal I.T. Workout

Before you start customizing an optimal I.T. Workout for yourself, think back to how you felt after your first I.T. Workout:

Were You Too Tired to Complete the Workout?

Be honest: Were you too tired to complete the workout? Or, did you finish but feel like a piece of overcooked hamburger by the end? That's okay; it happens sometimes. You're learning your limitations, so just think of it as a subtle clue that the intensity level needs adjusting. It's easy to fall into the "more is better" trap and take two steps up instead of just one. If you planned to do 10 reps but could only finish 8, chances are you were just pushing too hard and need to scale back the intensity next time. Another thing to consider is your level of fitness. Be honest: have you overestimated your fitness level? Are you truly ready for interval training? If not, don't sweat it. Just stick to aerobic exercise only for another month or so, slowly increasing the intensity or the distance covered, and then move on to the more challenging I.T. Workouts. Your body—and your medical insurance carrier—will thank you for it.

Did You Complete Your Workout with Ease?

If you completed your first I.T. Workout with ease, it means you didn't work hard enough! That's okay—it's not a bad idea to be on the conservative side when first start-ing out. Next time, nudge the intensity up a bit. Remember, it's those spikes in effort that enhance the I.T. effect, provided you don't cheat by compensating with fewer reps, shorter reps, or longer recovery intervals. Keep making adjustments until you have an optimal I.T. Workout—this usually takes from 2 to 4 sessions.

Did You Finish Tired but Able to Do More If You Had to?

If you finished tired but felt able to squeeze out a few more reps if you had to, congratulate yourself on a job well done. This is the optimal I.T. Workout, exactly how you want to feel after a hard training session.

Once you have achieved that perfectly balanced, fatiguing-but-not-exhausting I.T. Workout, it's time to shake things up and change it.

Huh? Why mess with success?

The thing is, the body doesn't improve without change—it adapts to whatever physical stress is heaped upon it, which is why the same workout that used to be so tough can eventually be done with greater ease. The ante needs to be upped again and again for progress to continue. Here's how to manipulate the four variables to make a stronger impact with your I.T. Workout.

Intensity

The intensity of each repetition is the first variable to adjust. The step up/one step method is an easy way for beginners to determine how much to increase or decrease the effort level, but there are other ways to do it, too.

Level

Level is useful with fixed exercise machines, such as treadmills, stationary bicycles, or stair climbers. Being able to crank up the level of resistance is a sure indicator of improved fitness.

Time

Time is a method that works best when the repetition is an unvarying, measurable distance, such as once around a track or a lap in the pool. Your ability to go at a progressively faster pace, completing each rep in less time, means your physical conditioning is getting better and better.

Feel

Feel is less black and white than other methods of gauging intensity, but it's the most flexible way and the one used most by elite athletes. You already use feel to some degree during your I.T. Workouts when you aim to finish up feeling tired but able to do a few more repetitions if you had to. Think of a runner doing repetitions at a stride pace. After doing enough interval training, she knows her abilities and can tell if she's running easy or hard. Being able to run more hard strides means she's improved her level of conditioning.

Self-assessment can be made less vague by using a number scale. You might say you did a rep at a "7 out of 10" pace, with 1 being very easy and 10 being your maximum effort. Or use a short word description to describe it, just as Joe Douglas, famed coach of the Santa Monica Track Club, uses with his runners: "easy" is a jog; "25 percent" is an average, natural pace; "fresh" is as fast as you can go while still able to hold a conversation; "good" is fast enough to cause fatigue; and "hard" is just short of going all out. Granted, "fresh" for a nationally ranked distance runner is going to be quite different than "fresh" for a 15-mile-a-week jogger, but it doesn't matter. Feel can take some getting used to, so experiment with it by recording the intensity of your reps in a training log, using whatever means of description works best for you.

Repetition Number

Once you have a better sense of how hard to push yourself, the next adjustment should be to the number of repetitions you do. This is the easiest variable of all to adjust—doing more reps is tougher than doing fewer, right? This is generally true—as long as each repetition is done at the same intensity, that is!

It's actually a good thing if you have only a limited amount of time to devote to each I.T. Workout. The body can only do so many quality repetitions before fatigue sets in. Push past fatigue and eventually the intensity level starts to free-fall and form gets sloppy (which increases the risk of injury). Pretty soon the whole workout is as flat as a purely aerobic workout, without the distinctive peaks and valleys of interval training. This defeats the whole purpose of the I.T. Workout, the goal of which is to become more fit in less time. For this reason, the core I.T. Workouts (outlined later in this book) generally limit the number of repetitions to no more than 50 to 60 percent more than in your baseline aerobic workout. Quality over quantity is always best for this particular workout.

If you're too wiped out to finish all the reps you planned to do, at least try to "put in the time" and finish out what's left of your workout at a slow, easy pace. Next time, do fewer reps and let your body fully adjust before adding any more. If things are too easy, try doing more repetitions next time.

Whatever you do, don't make the mistake of skipping the warm-up and cooldown in order to cram more reps into an I.T. Workout. The warm-up and cooldown go far in terms of injury prevention, and the handful of minutes it takes can avert future pain and wasted downtime. Don't sacrifice your health just to get in a few more reps.

Repetition Length

A repetition length of one minute (or a roughly equal distance) is a good starting point for three reasons:

- One minute of intense (but less than maximum-effort) exercise uses approximately 50 percent aerobic and 50 percent anaerobic energy.

- One minute is long enough to get into a rhythm at a certain pace, without feeling as if you're constantly starting and stopping.

- One minute is short enough to concentrate on sustaining a particular level of effort (something that gets harder with fatigue).

When should you change the length of your repetitions?

When you are trying to meet specific goals.

Longer repetitions (more than 1 minute and done at a slightly lower intensity) require more aerobic and less anaerobic energy to complete. They develop stamina—the ability to go faster for a longer distance or time. Shorter repetitions (about 30 seconds or so) are more anaerobic because they can be done at a higher level of effort. Shorter reps increase muscle power by developing more large muscle fibers, which come in handy when you're trying to beat your cycling buddies to the top of a steep hill.

You can also change repetition length whenever you want to add more spice to your workouts. Try mixing it up, doing long repetitions one session and short reps the next, to give your body better overall physical stamina and conditioning.

Interval

For most people, a rest interval of 2 minutes between 1-minute repetitions is ideal. It's long enough for lactic acid to clear out, yet not so long that muscles get overly cool (and thus more prone to injury). Remember, the interval largely dictates the intensity of the repetitions, so altering it can make an I.T. Workout geared more for stamina or for speed.

Basically, a shorter interval (one part repetition to one part interval) develops stamina, or aerobic power. Trying to complete high-intensity reps with a short recovery period means that a fair amount of lactic acid will still be hanging around, so you'll be working hard in an already fatigued state. That's good training for future competitions, especially those lasting less than 30 minutes. A longer interval (one part repetition to three parts interval) is best for those who want to do ultra-intense repetitions, because there's more time to rest and recover in between. This is the best way to develop the speed you'll need for that final, victorious sprint towards the finish line.

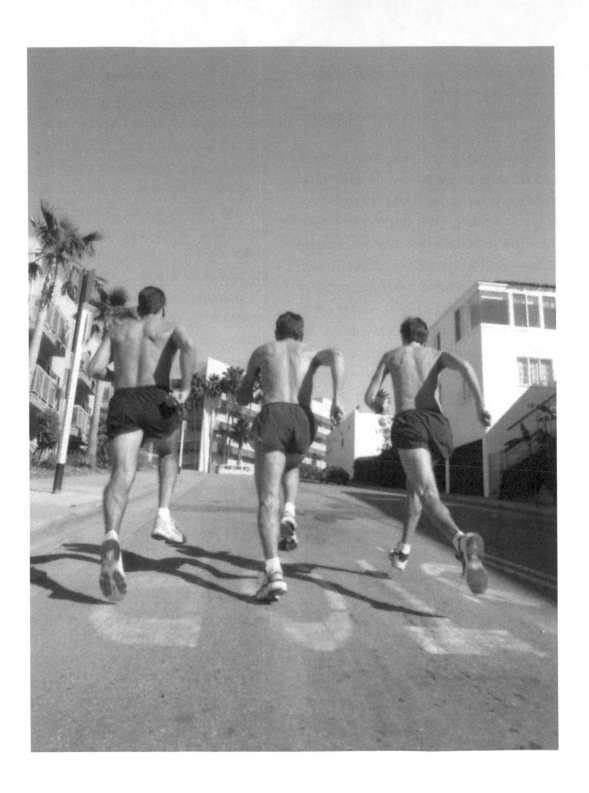

5

Putting It All Together: The Workouts

The I.T. Program uses a mix of three primary workouts:

- I.T. Workouts
- XL Workouts
- Active Rest Days

We will take a closer look at each one of these workouts and at ways to put them all together to create a challenging, results-oriented program tailored especially for you. At the end of this chapter are complete sample training regimens that incorporate these workouts for optimal fitness.

I.T. Workouts

After all this talk about I.T. Workouts, you're probably wondering:

How often should I do them?

After much trial and error by athletes and coaches, it seems that doing I.T. Workouts twice a week, with at least 48 hours between sessions, provides the best results for most people.

In the 1950s and 1960s, after the track world experienced its initial successes with interval training, an unabashed "more is better" attitude prevailed. Coaches pushed their athletes through daily (!) I.T. sessions, hoping to attain world-record fitness in world-record time. What they got instead was a bunch of exhausted, injured, and frustrated athletes. Later studies in the 1970s and 1980s revealed that doing such high-intensity exercise too frequently causes hormonal exhaustion. After a certain point the body is no longer able to adapt to the stresses placed upon it, and it basically crashes and burns.

These breakthrough revelations coincided with the "hard/easy" approach popularized by Bill Bowerman, the famous track coach of the University of Oregon (and one of the founding fathers of Nike). By alternating tough training sessions with easier recovery workouts, Bowerman and his successors produced dozens of world-class distance runners, including Steve Prefontaine. Today, the hard/easy approach is the most widely used method of training for elite athletes everywhere, and it provides the framework for the I.T. Program.

XL Workouts

An XL (Extra Long) Workout is simply your baseline aerobic workout done at a comfortable pace for, well, an extra-long time. The XL Workout is part of the I.T. Program for two excellent reasons:

- It burns fat.

- It builds mitochondria.

The longer an aerobic workout lasts, the more fat is used as a source of fuel. At the beginning of an aerobic workout, about two-thirds of the calories you burn are carbohydrates and one-third are fat. As time goes on, however, this ratio slowly changes; an hour into the workout, one-third of the calories burned are carbohydrates and two-thirds are fat. The longer you go, basically, the more fat you burn. That's not all. The longer an aerobic workout lasts, the more mitochondria are created. These help muscles use oxygen more efficiently, increasing the amount of exercise you can do aerobically.

Granted, this probably sounds pretty good. That's why some people are happy doing nothing but XL Workouts. You've probably seen these types at the gym, magazine in hand, strolling for what seems like forever on the treadmill you're impatiently waiting to use. They must feel they're getting some benefit, otherwise they wouldn't be doing it. But there are drawbacks to doing only this type of exercise. For one thing, it takes a lot of time. It also does nothing in terms of HGH production, it doesn't really work larger muscle fibers, and it doesn't do much to improve the ability to workout or compete at higher intensity levels. In the words of former world record holder and Olympic champion runner Sebastian Coe, "Long slow distance makes long slow runners." It's true. XL Workouts should be considered as just one element of a successful fitness program—to get maximum benefits you need to do I.T. Workouts and Active Rest Days as well. So limit XL Workouts to once a week, ideally at least 48 hours before or after an I.T. Workout.

Planning an XL Workout is easy. Just do your favorite aerobic exercise for a longer time than usual. Take it somewhat slower, so that you are comfortable and not pushing too hard, and just put in the time. The goal is to gradually increase this workout so that eventually it's 1½ to 2 times as long (measured by either distance or time) as your I.T. Workout, including warm-up and cooldown. For example, if your I.T. Workout in the pool takes 30 minutes, build up over time to make your XL Workout a slower, steady 45- to 60-minute swim. If you run 5 miles for your I.T. Workout, eventually you'll do 7.5 to 10 miles for your XL session.

An XL Workout can be a significant time commitment, no doubt about it. Many people like to schedule these longer sessions on weekends, when they have additional time to exercise. Trust us, it's time well spent. Once you start seeing the tangible results of your I.T. Program, you'll agree that XL Workouts are worth the effort.

Active Rest Days

An Active Rest Day is simply a light exercise session that maintains fitness and increases blood flow to tired muscles, aiding recovery between strenuous I.T. and XL Workouts. A good starting point is to do one-half to two-thirds of your baseline aerobic workout at about the same intensity (or slightly slower). If you normally walk on a treadmill for 30 minutes at 4 mph, for example, try doing 20 minutes at 3 to 4 mph on an Active Rest Day. Or use the time to do cross training with a different activity, if that's of interest.

The purpose of active rest is recovery—there's no benefit to making this workout any more challenging than it is. To be perfectly honest, if you can only manage to exercise 3 days a week, you should use the time for two I.T. Workouts and one

XL Workout (spacing them at least 48 hours apart), and skip the Active Rest Day completely. There will be ample rest the 4 days you don't work out!

Take a full day off once a week to give your body a break and to let it adapt to the exercise stress. When first starting the I.T. Program, these new, more challenging I.T. and XL Workouts may take longer to get used to than you would expect. Be flexible, and add additional Active Rest Days between harder workouts if necessary, or change an Active Rest Day into a full day off from exercise. If the quality of your harder workouts seems to be slipping, or if you feel overly tired or irritable or have trouble sleeping, you're probably pushing your body to do too much. Exercise should make you feel good. It should be fun—you'll never stick with it if it turns into a chore. So, be nice to yourself and don't feel guilty for taking some time off if your body needs more rest.

If you plan to exercise 6 days a week (which is ideal), the daily breakdown looks like this:

Day 1:   I.T. Workout

Day 2:   Active Rest Day

Day 3:   I.T. Workout

Day 4:   Day Off

Day 5:   XL Workout

Day 6:   Active Rest Day

Day 7:   Active Rest Day

Some people use an 8- or 9-day schedule, giving themselves 2 Active Rest Days or full days off after each hard workout. This doesn't produce results as quickly, but it's a good plan for older exercisers or those with time or energy constraints. For maximum gains, establish a schedule that works for you within 3 or 4 weeks of starting the I.T. Program, and then be consistent with it.

Progressing with the I.T. Program: The First 4 Weeks

Use the first month of the program to get used to the higher level of intensity. If it feels like the workouts are too hard or you have trouble completing them (even at a slightly slower pace), take an additional Active Rest Day or a full day off, and back off on the effort of your next I.T. Workout. If this doesn't resolve the situation, read the section on overtraining in the next chapter.

I.T. Workouts

Take a few sessions to figure out your optimal I.T. Workout. When it starts to feel easier, slightly increase the repetition intensity. Don't do any additional reps just yet—there's plenty of time for that later.

XL Workouts

Keep XL Workouts about 25 percent longer than your baseline aerobic workout. This allows your body to get used to a greater effort without pushing your endurance limits too hard.

Active Rest Days

On Active Rest Days, do about 50 to 70 percent of your baseline aerobic workout, at an easier intensity if necessary. The idea is recovery, so if you need to do less at first, by all means do so. Take a full day off at least once a week, 2 or 3 if you're still tired from the more strenuous workouts. (If you need more days off than this, tone down the intensity of your next I.T. Workout.) No matter how fabulous you feel, don't give in to the temptation to replace easy days with more I.T. and XL Workouts—this can lead to too much stress and potential for injury.

Moving Forward— Week 5 and Beyond

Once you hit week 5, it's time to move forward with your I.T. Program. By this time, you should notice that I.T. Workouts are getting easier, XL Workouts don't seem as long, and Active Rest Days are becoming even more appealing than lazing about the house. Time now to push ahead and further customize your I.T. Workouts to meet your individual needs. Here are a few things to keep in mind:

Increase Repetition Number or Repetition Intensity

Advance your I.T. Workouts by increasing either the repetition number or the repetition intensity. Do one or the other, but never both at the same time! If you increase the number of reps, add only 1 at a time and keep the upper limit about 50 to 75 percent above that of your optimal I.T. Workout. If you change the intensity, the sky's the limit for how challenging you can make it, but don't go nuts and exhaust yourself. Aim to feel tired but in control at the end of each workout. If you "hit a wall" with a higher intensity, try doing some reps at your previous intensity and some at the new, higher intensity during the same workout. Then slowly build up in subsequent workouts, doing more and more reps at the higher intensity level.

Change Repetition Length or Interval Length

To meet specific goals or to add variety, change the repetition length or the interval length. For example, do 1 short-rep/long-interval I.T. Workout and 1 long-rep/short-interval workout the same week. Adjusting these variables can be tricky since each one affects intensity, too. Track improvement by keeping notes on repetition number, repetition intensity, and interval length for each I.T. Workout you do. As you gain experience, you may want to try some alternative I.T. Workouts, such as those discussed at the end of this chapter. These workouts can be a nice break from routine and bring the same physiologic rewards as other I.T. Workouts when done with a similar high level of intensity.

Gradually Increase the XL Workout

Gradually increase the length of your XL Workout until it's 1½ to 2 times as long as the I.T. Workout, but no more than 2 hours. This workout takes considerably more time than the others, but the benefits are great.

Add Active Rest Days Whenever You Need Them

Always feel free to add Active Rest Days whenever you need them. If you start to need too many of these easy days, however, you're pushing too hard and need to adjust your I.T. and XL Workouts accordingly.

Don't Exercise More Than Six Days a Week

Exercising more than 6 days a week isn't a good idea. Your body needs time to rest and recover from all the physical stress it's being subjected to.

Take an Easy Week Every Four to Eight Weeks

Taking an easy week of Active Rest Days in place of your regular I.T. and XL Workouts won't sabotage your fitness—on the contrary, it will let you fully recover and avoid overtraining. Use it to cross train with a different activity if you wish, just for a change of pace. Aim to take an easy week every 4 to 8 weeks. Some people like to schedule these weeks during vacations or holidays, when a normal exercise routine is usually interrupted anyway.

Each Workout Is a Step Toward Greater Fitness

Remember that each workout is a step toward greater fitness. It's not possible to see improvement each and every workout. If it were, we'd all have a box filled with Olympic gold medals. Some days you'll be tired, or just "off." It happens to everyone—just do the best you can. If 1 or 2 workouts aren't so fabulous, back off a touch on the next session by decreasing either the repetition number or the intensity. If you have several sub-par workouts in a row, read up on motivation and goal setting in the next chapter. It might help get you out of your rut.

The Workouts

These workouts are the specific regimens that make up the I.T. Program. They're based on a 7-day cycle and are divided by activity (walking, running, cycling, swimming, and fixed exercise machines) for the first 4 weeks of the program and weeks 5 and beyond.

The I.T. Workouts are presented as either 30-minute or 60-minute sessions. If your intended workout time is longer or shorter, make adjustments accordingly.

All I.T. Workouts have the same repetition length, repetition number, and interval length for the first 4 weeks. You'll increase intensity as your fitness improves. In weeks 5 and beyond, we make recommendations for changing repetition number, intensity, and interval length. *Only adjust one variable at a time (you make the call on which one) and make changes gradually.* Just increase 1 rep at a time, for example, or slowly raise the intensity level or decrease the interval length over the course of several workouts.

All repetitions and intervals are based on time but can be easily converted to distance if you exercise in a measured setting (such as a track, marked trail, or pool, or if you use an odometer).

Some alternative I.T. Workout ideas can be found at the end of this chapter. Once you're past the first 4 weeks, shake up your program now and then by substituting one of these workouts in place of an I.T. session. You might even decide to make 1 or more of these alternative workouts a regular part of your I.T. Program.

Abbreviations used:

WU = warm-up (to be done at an easy, comfortable pace)

CD = cooldown (also at an easy pace)

I.T. = interval workout

XL = extra-long workout

AR = Active Rest Day (performed at intensity recommended or slightly lower intensity)

min = minute(s)

sec = second(s)

To make things easier, I.T. Workouts are written in this format:

repetition number x repetition length
and intensity/interval time

For instance, 8 1-minute reps done at level 6 with a 2-minute interval at level 2 is written as:

8 x 1-min at level 6/2-min at level 2

Walking

These schedules are for walkers doing 30 to 60 minutes of exercise 4 to 6 times a week. Intensity levels: slow walk, walk (your normal pace), jog, and run.

Weeks 1 to 4—30 Minutes

Day 1: I.T.
WU 10 min
5 x 1-min jog/2-min slow walk
CD 5 min

Day 2: AR 15–20-min walk

Day 3: I.T.
WU 10 min
5 x 1-min jog/2-min slow walk
CD 5 min

Day 4: Day off

Day 5: XL 37–38-min walk

Day 6: AR 15–20-min walk

Day 7: AR 15–20-min walk

Weeks 5 and Beyond—30 Minutes

Day 1: I.T.
WU 10 min
5 x 1-min jog/2-min slow walk
CD 5 min

Reps: increase to 8 x 1-min

Intensity: increase to run

Interval: decrease to 1-min

Day 2: AR 15–20-min walk

Day 3: I.T.
WU 5 min
4 x 2.5-min jog/2.5-min slow walk
CD 5 min

Reps: increase to 6 x 2.5-min

Intensity: increase to run

Interval: decrease to 1.5-min

Day 4: Day off

Day 5: XL increase gradually to 45–60-min walk

Day 6: AR 15–20-min walk

Day 7: AR 15–20-min walk

Weeks 1 to 4—60 minutes

Day 1: I.T.
WU 15–20 min
10 x 1-min jog/2-min slow walk
CD 5–10 min

Day 2: AR 30–40-min walk

Day 3: I.T.
WU 15–20 min
10 x 1-min jog/2-min slow walk
CD 5–10 min

Day 4: Day off

Day 5: XL 75-min walk

Day 6: AR 30–40-min walk

Day 7: AR 30–40-min walk

Weeks 5 and Beyond—60 minutes

Day 1: I.T.
WU 15–20 min
10 x 1-min jog/2-min slow walk
CD 5–10 min

Reps: increase to 15 x 1-min

Intensity: increase to run

Interval: decrease to 1-min

Day 2: AR 30–40-min walk

Day 3: I.T.
WU 10–15 min
5 x 3-min jog/3-min slow walk
CD 10 min

Reps: increase to 8 x 3-min

Intensity: increase to run

Interval: decrease to 2-min

Day 4: Day off

Day 5: XL increase gradually to 90–120-min walk

Day 6: AR 30–40-min walk

Day 7: AR 30–40-min walk

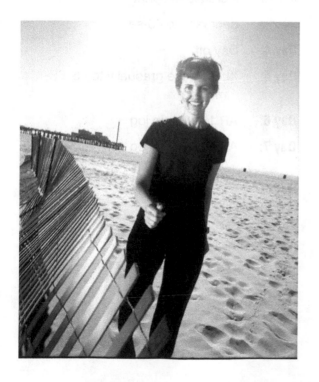

Jogging and Running

These workouts are for joggers and runners doing 30 to 60 minutes of continuous exercise 4 to 6 days a week. Intensity levels used are walk, jog (your normal pace), run, stride (a fast run), and sprint. If you are a more advanced runner, shift all intensities up a notch (substitute a 1-minute jog for a 1-minute walk, a 15-minute run for a 15-minute jog, a 2-minute stride for a 2-minute run).

Weeks 1 to 4—30 Minutes

Day 1: I.T.
WU 10 min
4 x 1-min run/2-min walk
CD 5 min

Day 2: AR 15–20-min jog

Day 3: I.T.
WU 10 min
4 x 1-min run/2-min walk
CD 5 min

Day 4: Day off

Day 5: XL 37–38-min jog

Day 6: AR 15–20-min jog

Day 7: AR 15–20-min jog

Weeks 5 and Beyond—30 Minutes

Day 1: I.T.
WU 5 min
4 x 2-min run/3-min walk
CD 5 min

Reps: increase to 7 x 2-min

Intensity: increase to stride

Interval: decrease to 2-min

Day 2: AR 15–20-min jog

Day 3: I.T.
WU 10 min
8 x 30-sec stride/1-min walk
CD 5 min

Reps: increase to 12 x 30-sec

Intensity: increase to sprint

Interval: decrease to 45-sec

Day 4: Day off

Day 5: XL increase gradually to 45–60-min jog

Day 6: AR 15–20-min jog

Day 7: AR 15–20-min jog

Weeks 1 to 4—60 Minutes

Day 1: I.T.
WU 15–20 min
8 x 1-min run/2-min walk
CD 5 min

Day 2: AR 30–40-min jog

Day 3: I.T
WU 15–20 min
8 x 1-min run/2-min walk
CD 5 min

Day 4: Day off

Day 5: XL 75-min jog

Day 6: AR 30–40-min jog

Day 7: AR 30–40-min jog

Weeks 5 and Beyond—60 Minutes

Day 1: I.T.
WU 15–20 min
6 x 2-min run/3-min walk
CD 10 min

Reps: increase to 8–10 x 2-min
Intensity: increase to stride
Interval: decrease to 2-min

Day 2: AR 30–40-min jog

Day 3: I.T.
WU 20 min
12 x 30-sec stride/1-min walk
CD 10 min

Reps: increase to 16–20 x 30-sec
Intensity: increase to sprint
Interval: decrease to 45-sec

Day 4: Day off

Day 5: XL gradually increase to 90–120-min jog

Day 6: AR 30–40-min jog

Day 7: AR 30–40-min jog

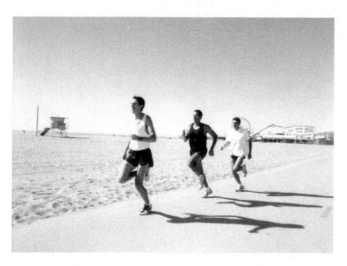

Cycling

These workouts are for cyclists who can ride continuously for 30 to 60 minutes in a low to middle gear. Pedaling rate (or rpm) should be kept constant at your natural rhythm. Intensity levels used: low gear, middle gear, and high gear. These gear levels are arbitrary; for instance, if you ride a ten-speed bicycle you may normally spin in the fourth gear (low-middle). If this is the case, then second gear will be low gear for you, middle gear may be sixth or seventh, high gear may be ninth or tenth. Adjust accordingly. Note: Those using stationary bicycles with varying levels of resistance may wish to refer to the Fixed Exercise Machine I.T. Program instead.

Weeks 1 to 4—30 Minutes

Day 1: I.T.
WU 5 min
5 x 1-min middle gear/2-min low gear
CD 5 min

Day 2: AR 15–20-min low-middle gear

Day 3: I.T.
WU 5 min
5 x 1-min middle gear/2-min low gear
CD 5 min

Day 4: Day off

Day 5: XL 37–38-min low-middle gear

Day 6: AR 15–20-min low-middle gear

Day 7: AR 15–20-min low-middle gear

Weeks 5 and Beyond—30 Minutes

Day 1: I.T.
WU 5 min
5 x 2-min middle gear/2-min low gear
CD 5 min

Reps: increase to 8 x 2-min

Intensity: increase to high gear

Interval: decrease to 1.5-min

Day 2: AR 15–20-min low-middle gear

Day 3: I.T.
WU 10 min
8 x 30-sec high gear/1-min low gear
CD 5 min

Reps: increase to 12 x 30-sec

Intensity: increase to 20 percent higher rpm in high gear

Interval: decrease to 45-sec

Day 4: Day off

Day 5: XL gradually increase to 45–60-min low-middle gear

Day 6: AR 15–20-min low-middle gear

Day 7: AR 15–20-min low-middle gear

Weeks 1 to 4—60 Minutes

Day 1: I.T.
WU 15–20 min
10 x 1-min middle gear/2-min
    low gear
CD 5 min

Day 2: AR 30–40-min low-middle gear

Day 3: I.T.
WU 15–20 min
10 x 1-min middle gear/2-min
    low gear
CD 5 min

Day 4: Day off

Day 5: XL 75-min low-middle gear

Day 6: AR 30–40-min low-middle gear

Day 7: AR 30–40-min low-middle gear

Weeks 5 and Beyond—60 Minutes

Day 1: I.T.
WU 15–20 min
6 x 3-min middle gear/3-min low
    gear
CD 5 min

Reps: increase to 10 x 3-min

Intensity: increase to high gear

Interval: decrease to 1.5-min

Day 2: AR 30–40-min low-middle gear

Day 3: I.T.
WU 15–20 min
12 x 30-sec high gear/1-min low
    gear
CD 10 min

Reps: increase to 20 x 30-sec

Intensity: increase to 20 percent higher
    rpm in high gear

Interval: decrease to 45-sec

Day 4: Day off

Day 5: XL gradually increase to 90–120-
    min low-middle gear

Day 6: AR 30–40-min low-middle gear

Day 7: AR 30–40-min low-middle gear

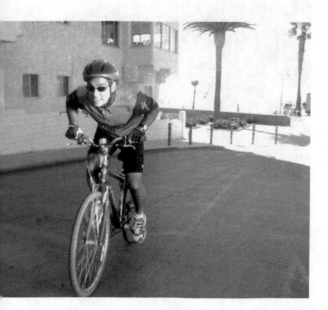

Swimming

These workouts are designed for swimmers who can do 30 to 60 minutes at a comfortable slow-to-medium pace. Intensity levels used: slow (turnover 20–30 percent slower than your baseline pace), medium (turnover 10–20 percent faster than baseline pace), fast (20–30 percent faster turnover), and sprint (30–40 percent faster turnover). These are rough estimates—remember that the goal is to finish each intense workout tired, but able to do a bit more if necessary.

There is one minor adjustment that is unique to swimmers: many pools have assigned lanes for various speeds, so varying your intensity during an I.T. Workout may not be possible. In this case, swim in the most appropriate lane for your repetition intensity, and spend the interval time resting at the end of the pool. Don't complete more repetitions than recommended. Instead, focus on maintaining a consistent level of intensity, so you are good and fatigued by the end of the workout.

Weeks 1 to 4—30 Minutes

Day 1: I.T.
WU 10 min
5 x 1-min medium/2-min slow
CD 5 min

Day 2: AR 15–20-min slow-medium

Day 3: I.T.
WU 10 min
5 x 1-min medium/2-min slow
CD 5 min

Day 4: Day off

Day 5: XL 37–38-min slow-medium

Day 6: AR 15–20-min slow-medium

Day 7: AR 15–20-min slow-medium

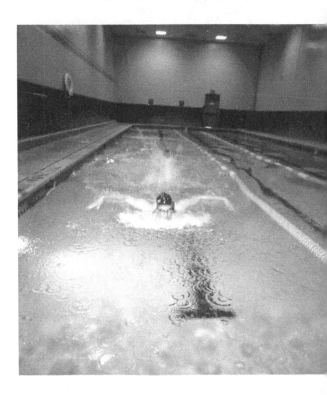

Weeks 5 and Beyond—30 Minutes

Day 1: I.T.
WU 5 min
4 x 2.5-min medium/2.5-min slow
CD 5 min

Reps: increase to 7 x 2.5-min

Intensity: increase to fast

Interval: decrease to 1.5-min

Day 2: AR 15–20-min slow-medium

Day 3: I.T.
WU 10 min
8 x 30-sec fast/1-min slow
CD 5 min

Reps: increase to 12 x 30-sec

Intensity: increase to sprint

Interval: decrease to 45-sec

Day 4: Day off

Day 5: XL gradually increase to 45–60-
min slow-medium

Day 6: AR 15–20-min slow-medium

Day 7: AR 15–20-min slow-medium

Weeks 1 to 4—60 Minutes

Day 1: I.T.
WU 15–20 min
10 x 1-min medium/2-min slow
CD 5–10 min

Day 2: AR 30–40-min slow-medium

Day 3: I.T.
WU 15–20 min
10 x 1-min medium/2-min slow
CD 5–10 min

Day 4: Day off

Day 5: XL 75-min slow-medium

Day 6: AR 30–40-min slow-medium

Day 7: AR 30–40-min slow-medium

Weeks 5 and Beyond—60 Minutes

Day 1: I.T.
WU 10–15 min
4 x 5-min medium/3.5-min slow
CD 5–10 min

Reps: increase to 7 x 5-min

Intensity: increase to fast

Interval: decrease to 2-min

Day 2: AR 30–40-min slow-medium

Day 3: I.T.
WU 20 min
12 x 30-sec fast/1-min slow
CD 10 min

Reps: increase to 20 x 30-sec

Intensity: increase to sprint

Interval: decrease to 45-sec

Day 4: Day off

Day 5: XL gradually increase to 90–120-
min slow-medium

Day 6: AR 30–40-min slow-medium

Day 7: AR 30–40-min slow-medium

Fixed Exercise Machines

These workouts are for exercisers who use stair climbers, stationary bikes, elliptical trainers, and cross-country ski machines for 30 to 60 minutes at a moderate baseline aerobic level 4 to 6 days a week. Intensity is measured by this baseline level (referred to here as "level X"), plus or minus additional levels. Because machine levels are not the same for all types of equipment, you may need to adjust the intensity so that you complete the more intense I.T. and XL Workouts tired but feeling like you could do a bit more if necessary. Remember to maintain the same rpm (on cycles, elliptical trainers, and cross-country ski machines) or step rate and depth (on stair climbers) that you would during a normal aerobic workout.

Weeks 1 to 4—30 Minutes

Day 1:   I.T.
WU 10 min
5 x 1-min level X+2/2-min level X-2
CD 5 min

Day 2:   AR 15–20-min level X

Day 3:   I.T.
WU 10 min
5 x 1-min level X+2/2-min level X-2
CD 5 min

Day 4:   Day off

Day 5:   XL 37–38-min level X

Day 6:   AR 15–20-min level X

Day 7:   AR 15–20-min level X

Weeks 5 and Beyond—30 Minutes

Day 1:   I.T.
WU 5 min
4 x 2.5-min level X+2/2.5-min level X-2
CD 5 min

Reps: increase to 7 x 2.5-min

Intensity: increase to X + 5

Interval: decrease to 1.5-min

Day 2:   AR 15–20-min level X

Day 3:   I.T.
WU 10 min
8 x 30-sec level X+4/1-min level X-2
CD 5 min

Reps: increase to 12 x 30-sec

Intensity: increase to X + 7

Interval: decrease to 45-sec

Day 4:   Day off

Day 5:   XL gradually increase to 45–60-min level X

Day 6:   AR 15–20-min level X

Day 7:   AR 15–20-min level X

Weeks 1 to 4—60 Minutes

Day 1: I.T.
WU 15–20 min
8–10 x 1-min level X+2/2-min
  level X-2
CD 10 min

Day 2: AR 30–40-min level X

Day 3: I.T.
WU 15–20 min
8–10 x 1-min level X+2/2-min
  level X-2
CD 10 min

Day 4: Day off

Day 5: XL 75-min level X

Day 6: AR 30–40-min level X

Day 7: AR 30–40-min level X

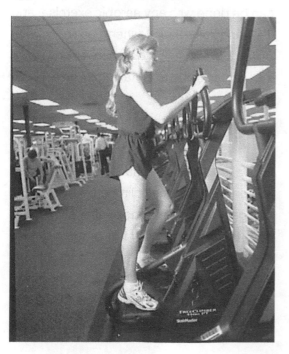

Weeks 5 and Beyond—60 Minutes

Day 1: I.T.
WU 20 min
5 x 3-min level X+2/3-min level
  X-2
CD 10 min

Day 2: AR 30–40-min level X

Day 3: I.T.
WU 20 min
12 x 30-sec level X+4/1-min level
  X-2
CD 15 min

Reps: increase to 20 x 30-sec

Intensity: increase to X + 7

Interval: decrease to 45-sec

Day 4: Day off

Day 5: XL gradually increase to 90–120-
min level X

Day 6: AR 30–40-min level X

Day 7: AR 30–40-min level X

Alternative I.T. Workouts

As you become more familiar with the concept and feel of interval training, you may wish to add a bit more spice to your program by occasionally doing one or more of the following alternative workouts in place of an I.T. session. These workouts offer an opportunity to learn more about your physical capabilities, and, more importantly, they're fun. Just remember to finish up feeling tired but still able to do a bit more.

Hills

Doing hills (or "gravity training," as we like to call it) is great for walkers, runners, and cyclists. Do an easy warm-up on the flats, then charge up a moderately steep hill at a good clip for 30 seconds to 2 minutes, then recover by descending slowly back to the bottom. Do enough of these repetitions and intervals to fill your intended workout time, then do a short cooldown. Another option is to put together a course with several different hills, some short, some long, pushing a bit as you climb to the top and backing off on the way down. If it's snowing or too slippery outside, do a hill workout on bleacher steps at a stadium or set a treadmill at an incline.

Fartlek

First of all, "fartlek" is a Swedish word that means "speed play," okay? It's a fun workout because you get to improvise as you go, doing bursts of speed for different distances with brief rests in between. After warming up, pick a random landmark—a tree some distance away or the end of the block—then just pick up the pace until you get there, slow down awhile to rest, then pick another landmark. It can be done with a stopwatch, too—just speed up for whatever amount of time you decide to do, rest a bit, and repeat. Keep at it until you have only enough gas left to do a little more, then do a short cooldown. Fartlek training can be done with any aerobic exercise, and it's especially useful when you're in unfamiliar surroundings or when easing back into speedwork after taking a little break from the program.

Group Exercise

Using fixed exercise machines—treadmills, stationary bikes, stair climbers—by yourself can get to be a real snooze after awhile. But now many gyms offer fun group exercise options such as "spinning"—a group cycling class guided by a coach who plays music and helps riders visualize things like cruising the plains or surging up a mountain pass in the Tour de France. Try one of these classes to help get you through. And, for any exercise activity, it's never a bad idea to find some training partners. Working out with other people is a great way to stay motivated, especially on hard days, and it helps make the time fly by.

AT (Anaerobic Threshold) Workouts

AT Workouts are specifically designed to train your body to manage lactic acid buildup over an extended period of time. After warming up, go for 15 to 20 minutes at a substantially higher level of effort than your baseline aerobic workout. Think of it as a 90 percent effort—you should be fairly tired two-thirds of the way through, and you should finish feeling like you could go on only if there were a gold medal on the line. Take a moment to catch your breath, then do a short cooldown. This type of workout is really taxing, so pace yourself and do it only occasionally.

Ladders and Pyramids

Varying repetition lengths can really jazz up an I.T. Workout. Try a "ladder," doing a 5-minute rep, then a 4-minute, then a 3-minute, and so on, making the interval equally long as each repetition. Or try a "pyramid": a 1-minute rep, then a 2-minute, then a 3-minute, then a 4-minute; back down to a 3-minute, a 2-minute, and a 1-minute; again using equally long intervals. Vary the intensity with the repetition length—ease back a bit for the longer reps, go faster for the shorter ones. Remember to warm up and cool down before and after these workouts, too.

Programmed Workouts

Many fixed exercise machines such as treadmills and stationary bikes have pre-programmed workouts that can vary intensity for you. Try to choose programs with a wide range of intensity levels and work to keep going at the same pace throughout.

Off-Road Workouts

Off-road workouts are a lot like fartlek workouts, the idea being to find more difficult terrain (such as a mountain bike trail, a beach, a hilly golf course, or an ocean or lake). Outside the controlled environment of a track or a flat road or a pool, the forces of nature conspire against good form and make things extra challenging. Pick up the intensity on the tougher sections—swim harder against the tide, run on the softer sand (where there's less traction and stability), lean hard on the pedals up a muddy trail. As always, work until you can only do a little more, then take an easy cooldown.

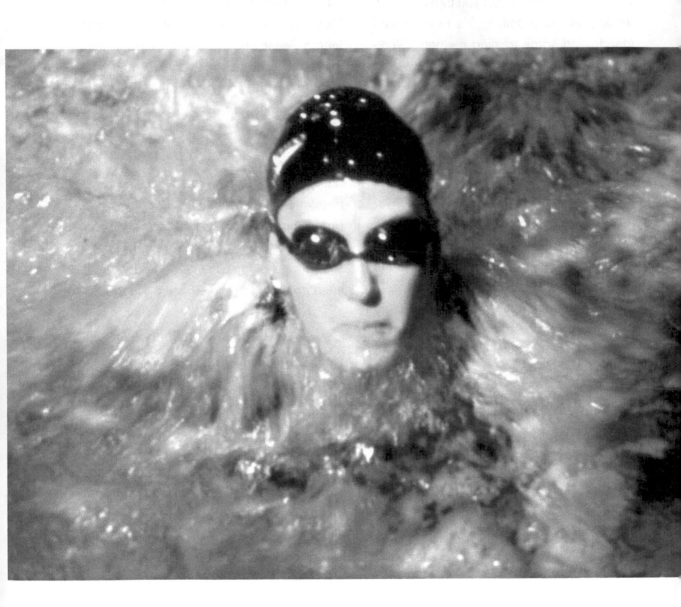

The Mental Edge: Motivation and Goal Setting

Millions of people pledge over and over every New Year's Eve to finally buckle down and get into shape. Why can't more people stick with it?

It isn't easy, that's why. In these hectic, over-scheduled times, exercising consistently is a real challenge, especially early in the morning when you're bleary-eyed with sleep or after work when dinner, friends, family, and television programs seem to take priority. Working out may do wonders for your physique and self-esteem and may even make you feel a bit superior to your friends and coworkers (come on, admit it) who can't muster the same discipline. But even the most dedicated competitive athletes peer out at the bleak predawn sky sometimes and wonder why on earth they aren't still snoozing in bed, like all the normal people.

The truth is that exercising regularly is not considered normal by a good portion of the general population. Anyone who has ever worked out early in the morning, or during a heat wave, or in the pouring rain has no doubt noticed a strange look or two. These tend to be either wistful (envious?) glances or expressions that seem to say, "I can't believe anyone is dumb enough to be out exercising in this." If you're devoted to attaining peak conditioning or even if you just want to make exercise a daily part of your life, you need to find a reliable way to stay motivated. It's hard, especially when you're exercising on your own, but if you believe enough in what you're doing, you'll somehow manage to crawl out of bed. The benefits of exercise make all the inconveniences worthwhile.

The encouraging thing is that if you've made it this far in this book, you probably already have what it takes to succeed. Nonetheless, your mind and your body may not always be on the same page when it comes to physical fitness, and at those times it helps to have some tricks to kick the two back into sync. Ask yourself the following:

- Are you motivated to work out most of the time, with only a few days a month on which you miss a workout or make a halfhearted effort because you don't feel like exercising?

- Do you find yourself dreading your next workout?

- Do you miss at least one scheduled workout a week?

Exercise should be a lifelong priority, so an occasional lack of willpower or a skipped workout is perfectly fine—even healthy—and nothing to beat yourself up about. What needs to be avoided at all costs is the attitude that not completing a workout somehow screws up all that's been previously accomplished and that continuing on is pointless. This is a silly but remarkably easy mental trap to fall into, and people on diets do it all the time. "I just blew my whole diet with that chocolate cookie, so today is a total loss and I may as well eat the rest of the box." Obviously, this defies all logic, but it's typical of the tricky nature of motivation. It's a head game, but you are in control. Every athlete at one time or another has substituted a nap or an evening with the remote control for a hard interval workout. Life is unpredictable and success comes through being flexible. So, unless you're training for the Olympic Trials, adapt your workout schedule to fit into your life. A day off here and there can give you a much-needed mental and physical break and let you come back with greater energy and enthusiasm next time.

The same thing holds true when you're on vacation or away from home. It's harder to exercise at the same intensity or for the same length of time in unfamiliar surroundings. So relax and enjoy yourself, and turn your workouts into an opportunity to explore. Try something different, such as running along the beach or sightseeing by bicycle, doing two-thirds of what you normally do, tops. Or, schedule a week of Active Rest Days to coincide with your travels. Even if you skip a session or two entirely, it won't throw your fitness program completely out of whack. Just plan to put in some quality workouts once you return to "real life."

Overtraining

If you find yourself dreading your next workout or miss at least one scheduled workout a week, there's a very good chance that you're doing too much. You're overtraining.

Sometimes the problem with motivation has less to do with overcoming guilt and inertia than it does with knowing when to stop exercising. Although we know that it's possible to exercise too much, overtraining is still a poorly understood physical phenomenon. The human mind, when properly motivated, can push the body to incredible lengths: climbing Mount Everest without oxygen; lifting a car to free a trapped person; running a marathon. But human physiology can adapt only so much and only at a given pace—otherwise, we would all be Olympians. This built-in ceiling

of adaptability is completely natural; it's the body's way of ensuring it doesn't run itself right into the ground. Take a few moments sometime to watch children at play. They run around and around until they are too tired to do it anymore, and then they stop and take a little nap. Unfortunately, hard-driving fitness enthusiasts and athletes often push right through this natural ceiling in pursuit of greater physical gains.

Over the course of a workout or a week of training, this pushing can lead to sore muscles and mild fatigue. This is expected to some degree—even sought after—in the course of the I.T. Program, because it's a sure sign that you're giving your body a thoroughly effective bout of exercise. I.T. and XL Workouts are never done on consecutive days because the schedule is designed to allow adequate physical (and mental) recovery between these more difficult sessions. Occasionally, you may overdo a workout and not recover in time for the next tough session—your working muscles might feel too sore or heavy or you might just lack the energy to complete the work. This is all part of learning your own limitations and is easily remedied with an extra day or two of Active Rest Day Workouts or a full day off.

There's a big difference, however, between merely overdoing it now and then and overtraining. Overtraining manifests itself in various ways, including:

- chronic fatigue

- lack of interest in working out

- irritability

- difficulty sleeping

- change in appetite

- lingering muscle soreness

A combination of these symptoms over a couple of weeks can lead to a mild case of exercise-induced depression, where the body tries to protect itself and replace depleted energy stores by refusing to adapt to any more physical stress. If you are willing to work towards greater fitness, you can't completely avoid the possibility of overtraining. The line between not enough and too much is extremely fine and changes over time as the body better adapts to stress. Almost everyone who follows a demanding fitness program and remains injury-free ends up in an exercise funk at some point. But good habits—such as proper diet, getting enough sleep, stretching, strength training, and cross training with other activities—can help you better tolerate the tougher workouts and recover from them more quickly.

World-class runners, swimmers, cyclists, and others at the highest levels of fitness tend to live like clocks, their daily lives scheduled with almost inhuman regularity—awake at a certain time, workout at a certain time, eat at a certain time, workout, rest, eat, sleep, repeat ad nauseum. Those T-shirts that say "Eat, Sleep, Run" aren't much of an exaggeration for these athletes, and it can be an exceedingly dull existence. Nonelite athletes aren't completely immune, either. It's amazingly easy to fall into a bad pattern of exercise addiction, where a growing obsession with working out begins to interfere with work or personal life. This is as much a problem as lack of motivation, because you not only burn out quickly, you also miss out on a lot of fun things in life. And that truly defeats the whole purpose of exercise, which is supposed to enhance these very things.

Small changes in your daily routine can help fend off the depressing, demoralizing effects of overtraining, which is why the I.T. Program includes a full week of Active Rest Days every 4 to 8 weeks. Such extended rest periods are an important element of this exercise plan and can save you the embarrassment of falling asleep during the eight o'clock reruns on TV. Can't beat that.

If you do find yourself getting irritable, tired, sore, and apathetic, or if workouts are becoming a real struggle, you're definitely pushing your physical envelope (or at least licking it). In some respects, this is a milestone to be celebrated. Given the increasingly sedentary nature of the American lifestyle these days, most people never even get a glimpse of their own physical capabilities, let alone embrace them. This is why cardiovascular disease is the number one killer in this country. You, on the other hand, have successfully managed to truly get out there on the edge.

It's a delicate balance. If the symptoms of overtraining last for more than 10 days or so, do the following:

Take Some Time Off from Exercise

Three to 5 exercise-free days can go far to alleviate overtraining. Depending on how burned out you are, this time will either feel like nirvana attained or an eternity in purgatory. Don't feel guilty about this time off—it's a mental health break as much as a physical one. Use the time to catch up on nonathletic activities, maybe going out for margaritas with friends, renting a stack of videotapes, or tossing sticks for your dog. Just don't think about working out.

Then Do a Week of Active Rest

Substitute Active Rest Days where you normally have an I.T. or XL workout for a full week. Take it easy and don't push yourself.

Resume Exercise at a Lower Intensity

Get back into the swing of working out by resuming exercise at a lower intensity level or with more frequent rest weeks (no more than one every 4th week). Following these steps will help get you back on track after a bout of overtraining and help you to look forward to a good, hard, sweaty workout again. Use the experience to better recognize the onset of overtraining in the future, so you can take steps early to avoid problems and keep moving toward your fitness goals.

If considerable fatigue persists, go back and repeat the rest and recovery formula above. If fatigue still persists after several weeks of rest and reduced training, it's a good idea to see a physician to rule out the possibility of a physical ailment.

Loss of Interest

Loss of interest is experienced by many athletes. Unless you thrive on Zenlike repetition, doing the same old exercise routine all the time eventually gets to be, well, routine. If you feel good physically but find yourself sleepwalking with boredom through workouts, you obviously need to jazz things up to stay motivated. Here's how using the I.T. Program can help:

I.T. Workouts Go More Quickly

Interval Training Workouts seem to pass by more quickly. The varied effort level required for interval training relieves the monotony common to purely aerobic workouts.

I.T. Workouts Offer Variety

Each I.T. Workout can be structured in various ways so you are always doing something new and interesting. Within a single training week, you might do a workout with longer but fewer repetitions (e.g., 5 hard reps lasting 2 minutes) or do more reps for a shorter time (e.g., 15 reps that last 30 seconds). This not only breaks up routine, it also lets you emphasize the aerobic system one time, the anaerobic system the next.

XL Workouts Build a Solid Aerobic Base

XL Workouts build up endurance and a solid aerobic base and also provide a break from the more intense I.T. sessions.

The I.T. Program Gets Results

There are few things more motivating than seeing and feeling the fruit of your consid-erable labors. The I.T. Program gets results. You'll see improvement in the quality and quantity of individual workouts, be it in performing more high-intensity repetitions with less effort or in having more than enough endurance to go for an especially challenging XL Workout.

And there are still other ways to help keep up your interest:

Make Your Workouts a Habit

Successful exercisers make workouts a habit. Try to exercise at the same time of day and under similar conditions as often as possible. Think of your workouts as scheduled appointments and stick to 'em. Motivation is a psychological issue as much as it is a physical one, and if you train your mind and body to anticipate exercise at a certain time and place each day, it becomes almost second nature. You not only are prepared to work, you look forward to it and may even feel slightly out of sorts when you can't squeeze in a workout. It's a chance to devote time solely to yourself, away from the pressures of career, kids, e-mail, and phones. As noted before, however, be careful not to allow your habit to become too rigid. You might find yourself in a psychological slump if something prevents you from sticking to your workout schedule. This is a common experience for many athletes who suffer an injury and have to take a lengthy break from exercise.

Cross Train

Cross training with other sports and physical activities does wonders to break up the monotony of the "same-old, same-old," and it aids overall conditioning by calling into use different muscles and movements. (See Chapter 7 for tips on incorporating cross training into your program.)

Exercise with Others

Exercising with a friend or a group of others, even on a sporadic basis, can be a fun and sociable thing to do. The mere fact that you have a standing commitment to show up—which is half the battle on days when you're in a slump and have zero interest in working out—is reason enough to enlist the support of others. There's something about being surrounded by like-minded individuals that truly hones the motivational edge. They can provide encouragement and even an added spark of friendly competition, both of which can help push you to perform better than ever.

There are a few things to keep in mind, however. Limit your sessions with others to no more than 3 times a week, perhaps only on days scheduled for harder workouts.

This allows you to recover more fully between hard exercise sessions, because you're free to do your Active Rest Workouts at your own easy pace. Another thing to remember is that exercising with someone else doesn't mean you have to compete with each other or even do the same workout. Focus on doing what's right for you and coordinate things so that you and your buddy finish about the same time. It's rare for two individuals to be at identical fitness levels, so don't worry if you do a little more or less than the other guy. When we do Interval Training Workouts at the track with friends, whoever is less fit runs half or two-thirds of each repetition with the stronger runner, then takes a bit longer rest interval as the other completes the full repetition. Works for us.

Listen to Music (or Don't)

Listening to music is a crucial tool for some people to maintain motivation when exercising. At big competitions, many athletes can be found off in a corner somewhere with a set of headphones, either "psyching up" or trying to relax before their event with their favorite tunes. Music can make time pass more enjoyably, especially during some of those seemingly endless XL Workouts, and can make gutting through those last few I.T. repetitions a little easier, too. You can even make your own tapes or CDs to play during workouts, to use for a pre-race energy boost, or to wind down after a particularly grueling session. But it's a matter of individual taste. There are an equal number of purists out there who like things quiet when they work out and find that music distracts them from the feedback provided by their own bodies. One of the authors of this book is squarely in this latter camp; the other is just as stubborn about the advantages of the former. Do whatever works for you! Those music lovers who exercise out-of-doors wearing personal stereos need to be extra-vigilant of vehicle and pedestrian traffic, and women should also be hyperaware of their surroundings. If you find yourself getting into unfamiliar territory, switch off the music and keep your ears open to what's going on around you instead. Personal safety is the most important thing.

Keep a Training Log

We swear by keeping a training log and so do countless other athletes. Since many of us can't recall what we had for breakfast, let alone what we did for a workout weeks ago, a training log is invaluable to chart how far you've come, and what works and what doesn't work. Flipping through an old training log can be a truly satisfying experience, as it tells you just how much you've accomplished over time. Set aside a special notebook or make daily notations on a calendar to record what you did for your workout, as well as how you felt that day—several days of "feel great" sessions obviously indicate that training is optimal, while multiple "blah" entries (when you're tired, sluggish, or apathetic) point towards possible overtraining. Being able to see this at a glance can help nip problems in the bud—before they turn into chronic issues. Some people also record their diet or their resting pulse rate, taken a few minutes after waking up in the morning (a continuously elevated resting heart rate can indicate overtraining, a good sign to back off a bit on workouts). There's a sample training log at the back of this book that can be photocopied and used to track your own progress, and there are several versions you can buy at bookstores or sporting goods shops. A simple notebook with hand-drawn columns works just as well.

Put On Your Shoes

Sometimes the hardest part of working out can be just overcoming inertia. On days when you have zero interest in working out, focus on putting on your shoes, your swimsuit, or loading the bike into the car—the battle's half won right there. Then tell yourself to do only the first 5 minutes of your workout. Usually, once you start moving, you're likely to continue. Hey, it works for us. If you still feel awful after 5 minutes, bag the workout and take a day off.

Problems with Goal Setting

Working toward a goal is psychologically easier than working without one. But since many of us haven't a clue as to what we are truly capable of, setting an appropriate goal can present a bit of a problem—or two problems, as it usually turns out.

Overly High Expectations

Some folks are so pumped up at the prospect of a new workout program that they succumb to delusions of grandeur. It's admirable to think big, but we're all limited by genetics and by our many "real-life" responsibilities, so beware of overly high expectations. To be perfectly honest, many elite athletes are genetic freaks (in the best possible sense, of course) and have natural abilities that the rest of us just plain don't have—and never will. Most of us aren't able to train for sub–4-minute miles while juggling a full-time career or medical school (as Dr. Roger Bannister somehow managed to do). Attempting to do so will only result in overtraining, discouragement, frustration, or injury.

Nonexistent Expectations

The antithesis of the Walter Mitty–like behavior described above is to carry on without any expectations whatsoever. A lackluster approach to exercise, such as vaguely vowing to get into shape, can be just as counterproductive as setting overly ambitious goals. What will motivate you to put your shoes on when it's pouring rain outside? When there's a pepperoni pizza in the freezer? When the big game is playing on TV?

It might help to think of each workout as a deposit into a savings account. It's easier to make deposits when you are saving up for something specific—like a trip to Tuscany or a new BMW—isn't it? Some athletes begin training for a specific race up to 9 months in advance. These folks obviously aren't pushing themselves with undefined, nebulous goals. They know exactly what they want and carefully plan every step it's going to take for them to get there. That's strong goal orientation, and it can do wonders for your motivation, too.

Realistic goal setting, done with both feet planted squarely on terra firma, can be the best motivational tool around. Here are a few guidelines to help you create some attainable goals:

Think of the Big Picture

Start out by considering the big picture— why are you exercising? Is it to increase fitness to lose weight or to increase your overall sense of well being? Use this fundamental reason to provide a framework for your I.T. Program.

Then Think Specifics

Once you establish exactly why you're working out, think specifics and set your sights on a clear goal. It may be an athletic goal (such as finishing a 10K or hiking to the top of a nearby mountain) or it may be more aesthetically oriented (fitting into your college jeans again). Then find something to visually remind you of the goal, put it where you can see it everyday, and get to work.

Be Realistic!

As with New Year's resolutions, it can be self-defeating to be overly ambitious. Be realistic and set attainable goals that you can feel good about achieving.

Small Steps Work Best

It works best to break your goal into achievable steps (or "easily digestible chunks," as a friend of ours likes to put it). Jog a mile, then 2, then 3, before tackling a 5K race. Hopefully, once you accomplish a particular goal, you'll be pumped up enough to set a new, more ambitious goal. Perhaps a 10K? But first....

Reward Yourself

Ah, the best part. Reward yourself. Savor the moment before rushing off on yet another quest. Take a deep breath and tell yourself how wonderful you are, enjoy a tall, cool one after a race with your friends, buy a devastating dress after dropping those last 10 pounds. Maybe even treat yourself to a little vacation. Joseph went to Hawaii after qualifying for the Olympic Trials with a 2:18 marathon (and basically just waddled from the pool to the buffet table and back for a week). Rest and recover! Bask in your achievement awhile, then move on to the next lofty goal on your list.

Your Notes:

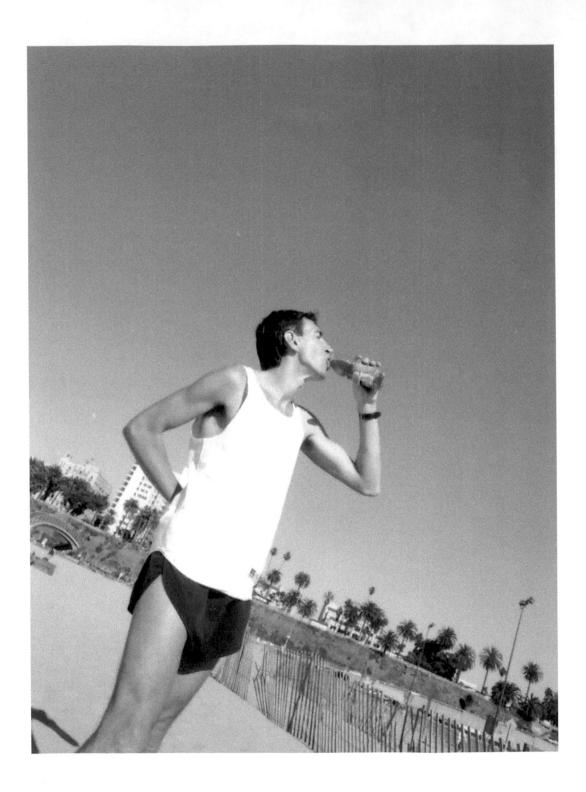

Beyond I.T.— Diet, Strength Training, Cross Training, Stretching, and Injury Prevention

The I.T. Program is an efficient, scientifically and clinically proven method of increasing fitness, burning calories, building more lean muscle mass, and greatly improving your cardiovascular system function. As a stand-alone program it definitely produces results.

But is the I.T. Program enough?

You can make the I.T. Program's results even more dramatic by incorporating into it better nutrition, strength training, cross training, stretching, and injury prevention measures. Whole books have been written about each of these topics by experts in their particular fields (which, in these areas at least, we readily admit we are not). But for the purpose of this book, some comments on these subjects from an athlete's perspective and an overview of how each can accentuate the I.T. Program may be of interest to you.

Diet

People love to talk about their latest diet. The Zone Diet, the Pritikin Diet, the Grapefruit Diet, the Cabbage Soup Diet (we're not making this up) are just a few. There's usually a gimmick of some sort involved: counting points, measuring food portions, eating certain food combinations, eating only at certain times of day. And, the people who dream up these gimmicks are, of course, making a fortune.

Perhaps you've experienced some success yourself with a fad diet at one time or another. Why is this?

It's because any diet has the potential to work, initially, simply because followers are thinking about what they put into their mouths.

People who are conscious of their eating habits tend to eat less. But any diet that withholds adequate calories and nutrients or eliminates whole food groups or is too cumbersome to keep up on a long-term basis is doomed to failure. Millions of overweight people all too often discover this for themselves.

The high-intensity nature of the I.T. Program calls for some special nutritional con-

siderations, and you might actually need to eat more calories, not less, to maintain a healthy weight. Your body needs fuel for peak performance. Dramatic changes to your diet probably aren't necessary—just a tweak here and there can really make a difference. If you think your eating habits could use a more extensive overhaul, be sure to consult a nutritionist or physician. Here are a few more things to keep in mind next time the conversation swings around to dieting issues:

A Calorie Is a Calorie

A calorie is a calorie. The body makes no distinction between 500 calories worth of chocolate cupcakes and 500 calories of carrot sticks; all it sees is 500 units of stored energy. The body uses whatever happens to be lying around. This isn't to say that a 100-percent-protein diet or a 100-percent-carbohydrate diet or a 100-percent-fat diet would all affect the body the same way. Each of these energy sources has its place: protein is needed to build muscle and other tissues; carbohydrates are a main fuel source for the brain and working muscles; fat serves as an efficient source of calories to all systems. This is why experts always harp on the need to have a well-balanced diet with a variety of foods from all three sources.

There's No Secret to Long-Term Weight Loss

To lose weight you need to burn more calories than you take in. That's it. Period. The only natural ways to create this calorie deficit are to eat less, exercise more, or do a combination of both. Studies show that people doing the combo plan lose weight faster and are more successful at keeping it off—so eat sensibly and exercise regularly.

Calories Are Fuel for Your Body

Calories provide fuel for your body, a good thing for anyone who exercises hard. You won't find many elite athletes on wacky, ultra-restrictive diets. They treat their bodies like machines, fueling them well to keep things operating at peak levels. Eat when you're genuinely hungry, because that's a signal that you're running low on energy. For the first few weeks of the I.T. Program, you may be hungrier than usual, but it'll level out soon enough. Does all that hard exercise give you free rein to mainline junk food or chow down sumo wrestler–sized portions? Nope. Instead, add a bit more to your regular meals or have nutritious mini meals, perhaps every 3 or 4 hours, and stop eating when you aren't hungry anymore. It seems ridiculously easy, but it may take time to adjust to this sort of natural eating.

Athletes Need Carbohydrates

Skimping on daily carbohydrate intake can actually hinder your I.T. Program. Athletes need them. You burn carbs and some fat during aerobic workouts, but for harder, anaerobic sessions the primary fuel comes from carbohydrates. And, since the body's limited glycogen (carbohydrate) stores become depleted very quickly, it's crucial to eat enough carbs when you start doing speedwork. Without them, you'll eventually "bonk" and not have an ounce of "umph" left in you to gut it out to the finish line. The same effect can also occur over a period of days or weeks, as glycogen stores are used up faster than they're replaced. So eat carbs, just don't go overboard with them—too many carbohydrates can cause blood sugar levels to swing.

Keep It Simple

Complicated, rigid diet plans are a waste of time. To improve eating habits, keep it simple—isolate one unhealthy habit at a time and make changes there. Instead of a pint of ice cream for dessert every night, say, have it once a week, or switch to frozen yogurt. Or vow to quit eating on autopilot, mindlessly plowing through whole bags of chips or cookies in front of the TV. Add more fruits, veggies, and grains so your daily diet is about 60 percent carbohydrate, 15 percent protein, and 25 percent fat. Focus on doing consistent, high-quality I.T. Workouts and forget about obsessively counting calories.

Q. How does metabolism work?

Metabolism works like this: the body's basic unit of energy is the much-maligned calorie (a "kilocalorie," technically, but hardly anyone calls it that). Each gram of carbohydrate provides 4 calories; each gram of protein 4 calories; and each gram of fat provides 9 calories. To gain a single pound you need to eat 3,500 more calories than your body uses, and to lose a pound you have to burn those same 3,500 calories off. No wonder losing weight is so difficult!

What a lot of people don't know is that each gram of stored carbohydrate retains 9 grams of water, while protein and fat store little or no water. This is why those popular high protein/low carb diets produce such amazing results the first few weeks. Basically, when few carbohydrates are eaten, the body turns to stored carbs for energy, and that retained water is released and flushed out of the system. The weight lost isn't fat—it's mostly water weight. While preparing for a marathon, Joseph avoided carbohydrates for 3 days to deplete glyco-gen stores as part of a carbo-loading regimen. In that brief time, his weight dropped from 154 to 147 pounds, despite his training only half as much as usual. But then, after 3 days of eating carbs again, he was back at his usual weight again. Did he somehow manage to lose and then regain almost 25,000 calories in 6 days? Of course not. It was all water weight.

Eating too much protein can cause irritability and fatigue because the brain—which feeds primarily on carbohydrates—isn't getting the calories it needs to maintain its everyday functions. High-protein diets are tough on the kidneys and make for rather limited dining options, too, so it's probably for the best that most people can't stick to this sort of eating for very long. Of course, some protein is necessary, especially for people who do higher intensity exercise. A little common sense and moderation go a long way.

Is it possible to manipulate metabolism with fad diets? Sure, but only briefly. The body eventually fights off any self-imposed starvation by going into an energy-saving mode, making you too sluggish to squander precious calories exercising. It's a natural survival mechanism, and, judging by the number of glassy-eyed couch potatoes out there, it works really, really well. Crafty schemes to drop weight fast tend to backfire with the dreaded yo-yo effect: metabolism drops until the body eventually revolts and demands to chow down in an effort to shore up against any future "famines." The net result is weight gain. So just use your common sense. It's not smart to mess with Mother Nature.

Q. What should I eat before, during, and after an I.T. or XL workout?

Eating Pre-Workout

Hard exercise temporarily slows down your digestion, which explains why a cheeseburger sits in your stomach like a rock when you go running right after lunch. But doing a workout on a completely empty stomach isn't too smart either, as it can leave you hypoglycemic, frazzled, and unmotivated. Many athletes find that exercising when they're slightly hungry seems to work best—there's not much sloshing around inside, and the physical exertion usually releases enough glucose and fat into the bloodstream that they can make it through the session. If you must eat, and plan to train in less than an hour, a sports drink packing easy-to-digest carbs might do the trick. If you want something more, make sure it's light and mostly carbohy-

Q. Do I need to take vitamins or supplements?

Taking a simple multivitamin is useful for anyone whose diet isn't as balanced as it could be, as well as for teenagers, vegetarians and vegans, and pregnant women. Some experts say nutrients should ideally come only from whole foods, but unless you want to nosh on spinach all day long, it's just more practical to pop a vitamin to fill in nutritional gaps. More isn't necessarily better when it comes to vitamins, so take the recommended dosage and leave it at that. Another thing: vitamins are vitamins, so opt for the cheaper generic versions over expensive name brands. It's all the same on the inside, just slicker packaging and marketing on the outside.

drate, so you won't be running on empty but can still exercise comfortably. (A piece of toast with a thin spread of peanut butter or a sports drink or half a banana should do it.) Some people who exercise first thing in the morning find that having a midnight snack carries them through their workout nicely. Try to avoid fatty foods before a workout—they're a chore to digest and leave you feeling sluggish. Energy bars? There are dozens out there to pick and choose from, but to be honest, many elite athletes never eat them. They pack up to 300 calories and more protein than you need in an entire day and don't do anything magical for your body or your performance, either. Some taste like chalk and others are really candy bars in disguise. But if you like them, they're fine for a pre-workout snack.

Eating During a Workout

You won't want to eat anything during an I.T. Workout, but it's a different story with the longer XL sessions. There's nothing worse than being at the turnaround point of a 40-mile-loop bike ride and feeling too dehydrated or hypoglycemic to get all the way back home. Make sure you tote along a bottle of water or diluted fruit juice or a sports drink (8 ounces worth for every 20 minutes of exercise) and a small, easily absorbed snack such as raisins or a banana. Research shows that simple carbohydrates taken in during a long bout of exercise are used as a source of energy by working muscles, preserving glycogen (carbohydrate) stores. If you're setting off for a really long endurance workout, particularly if it's a warm day, bring a light, high-carb, salty snack (such as pretzels or chips) to replace sodium lost in sweat.

Eating Post-Workout

Time to chug and chow. Research shows that having a simple high-carb snack either immediately after or 2 hours after an intense workout is the best way to replace depleted glycogen stores. Rehydrating is important too, and few things quench thirst better than plain old water. Later on, you'll probably be ravenous and ready to tear the door off the refrigerator. Have something with enough calories to replace whatever you burned off. Many athletes stick to carbo-junkie staples such as pasta, rice cakes, bagels, pretzels, and bread for their post-workout meals. These are fine, but add some fat so you won't be hungry again for awhile. Toss in some fruit and vegetables too; they contain antioxidants that help fend off muscle damage and injury.

Hydration "Do"s and "Don't"s

Coaches and trainers all over the world make the same complaint about their elite athletes: they're chronically dehydrated. You probably are too. The body is 50 to 65 percent water and needs to be constantly topped off. Exercising hard increases fluid loss since water is excreted as sweat to cool things down. Dehydration causes the blood to thicken and forces the heart to work harder. It slows the delivery of oxygen and nutrients to the muscles and can leave you sluggish and unable to concentrate. It also lowers your ability to tolerate lactic acid, which makes you feel exhausted faster. It's just bad all around, so drink up! If possible, take in at least 4 to 8 ounces of fluid every 15 to 20 minutes when exercising hard, more if it's a hot day. Don't wait until you're thirsty—that's a sign you're already dehydrated. Good rules of thumb: drink twice as much as it takes to quench your thirst; drink enough that your urine is clear or light yellow in color; keep caffeinated drinks and alcohol to a minimum (they're dehydrating); and follow every workout with at least 24 ounces of water or a sports drink. Which sports drink is best? Here's a quick rundown.

Regular Sports Drinks

Sports drinks are great to swig down before or during a workout and may even be a better option than water during long, hot endurance sessions. All sports drinks include electrolytes such as sodium and potassium, which are important whenever you sweat heavily.

Fitness Water

Tastier than plain water, fitness waters are flavored drinks with 10 to 25 calories per 8-ounce bottle, a touch of sodium and potassium, and even a few vitamins, perfect for workouts lasting less than an hour when you don't need the high calories of a sports drink. Watered-down fruit juice works well too.

Recovery Drinks

High-calorie recovery drinks are ideal for before or after exercise when a good boost of carbohydrates (about 160 to 240 calories per 8-ounce bottle) comes in handy. Use them in place of solid food before a hard workout or as a snack afterward to tie you over until chow time.

Strength Training

Strength training is an important part of the I.T. Program. Any workout program that focuses primarily on cardiovascular development can leave certain muscle groups more or less neglected. You've probably seen how distance runners have well-developed leg muscles with comparatively scrawny upper bodies, with swimmers just the reverse. To some degree, this can actually offer some competitive advantage. In the grueling Tour de France, for example, having heavily muscled legs is a given, but a heavily muscled upper body only serves as extra weight to haul up steep mountain climbs. When Lance Armstrong returned to the Tour pounds lighter after a long bout of chemotherapy, his leaner upper body was a factor that helped propel him to the winner's podium.

For those of you who aren't training for the Tour (yet), it's a good idea to add strength training to your I.T. Program to strike a balance between the primarily used "I.T. muscles" and the rest of the body. Strength training offers several advantages.

Injury prevention—Maintaining a balance between opposing muscle groups can prevent injury by protecting against a "weak link" failure.

Muscle adaptation—Much like an I.T. Workout, intense strength work (that is, working to muscle failure) causes muscle adaptation, a higher metabolic rate, and greater strength.

A completed package—A full-body strengthening regimen develops a more complete package by increasing overall body fitness, improving the physique, and boosting self-image.

Strength training offers benefits extending beyond mere fitness, such as building up bone mass to stave off osteoporosis in women. All that's needed are a few pieces of equipment and a handful of extra minutes a week. You can give yourself an in-depth crash course on strength training by consulting any one of the many books and magazines currently out there on the subject. For now, here are a few thoughts to get you started:

Strength Training Should Supplement the I.T. Program

Strength training should be a supplement to the I.T. Program. If your time is too crunched to handle both strength training and the I.T. Program, focus energy on the latter. However, recent studies suggest that nearly as much benefit can be had from a single set of weight repetitions as from multiple sets, so it may be possible to squeeze in some training after all. You won't end up looking like Arnold Schwarzenegger doing this sort of abbreviated weight routine, but in a pinch, one set might do the trick.

Strength Train 2 to 3 Days a Week

Most people do strength work on Active Rest Days, 2 to 3 days a week, when their shorter workout allows extra time to lift weights. Any time is fine; the goal is merely to get it done. Allow at least a full day between sessions to give muscles a chance to recover and rebuild.

Focus on Neglected Muscle Groups

Don't overburden yourself with dozens of exercises. Instead, focus on neglected muscle groups. Otherwise, you'll just spend more time in the gym, cutting in on time better devoted to cardiovascular training. A handful of well-selected exercises that can be done quickly and consistently will suffice.

Do Minimal Strength Training for I.T. Muscles

Many athletes think strengthening their primary movers (the main muscles used for a given activity, such as calf muscles for running) provides added power and speed. There may be some merit to this, but usually these muscles are already working hard just doing the I.T. Program and need minimal additional strengthening. At least for the first few months of more intense workouts, concentrate only on more neglected muscle groups, such as upper body muscles for walkers, runners, cyclists, and people who use stair climbers and similar machines.

Keep a Written Log

Keep track of your strength training with a written log, just as you do for your other I.T. Program workouts. Include the number of sets, number of reps, and amount of weight lifted for each exercise. At the very least, the log will remind you where to set the weight next time you lift; even better, it will show you how much stronger you are getting. Nothing beats tangible evidence of improvement for motivation.

Do Alternative Exercises

They're just what they say they are—alternative exercises to your regular strength-training regimen. Leave the dumbbells in the closet and use your own body weight or other stuff instead. Do slow push-ups with good form to isolate the chest, shoulders, and triceps. Use family-sized cans of ravioli or buckets or plastic jugs filled with water, sand, or dirt—anything that weighs a few pounds. Take advantage of the workout stations found in some public parks or recreation areas. Do tricep dips on a chair or bench, climb a rope, play with rubber resistance bands, haul rocks uphill, or bench-press the dog. The idea is to add some variety and fun to what can sometimes be rather dull work. Some suggestions are listed below.

Mix It Up

Add variety by mixing things up a bit. You can do your strength-training exercises as straight sets (doing 1 to 3 sets of each exercise before moving on to the next), as circuits (doing 1 set of several different exercises, then repeating), or as supersets (doing 1 set each of two consecutive exercises, such as chest/back or biceps/triceps, and then resting).

With the exception of swimming, most activities involved with the I.T. Program focus on leg muscles, so your strength training should emphasize upper body and trunk work. Here's a sample workout week for someone who has basic strength-training experience. If you're just starting out, choose lighter weights than you think you can handle and do just one set of each exercise. Slowly adjust the weight over the course of a few sessions until you reach muscle failure—when you can't lift the weight anymore. This is your baseline—it's what you're able to lift at your weakest and puniest! From here on out, you're only going to get stronger.

Day 1: 1–3 sets of 10–12 repetitions of strength exercises (up to 15 if advanced)

Endurance: 1–3 sets of 10–25 sit-ups and dead lifts

Day 3: 2–3 sets of 3–6 repetitions of strength exercises with slightly heavier weights

Power: weight (the first set should be a warm-up set with lighter weights)

1–3 sets of 10–25 sit-ups and dead lifts

Day 5: alternative exercises

Suggested strength exercises for a fast but thorough upper body workout are described and pictured on the following pages.

Barbell or Dumbbell Bench Press

Lie face up on a flat bench holding a barbell or two dumbbells over the middle of your chest at arm's length, palms facing forward. Lower the weights until they are just outside your shoulders. Return to the starting position and repeat. Muscles emphasized are the pectoralis major, anterior deltoids, and triceps.

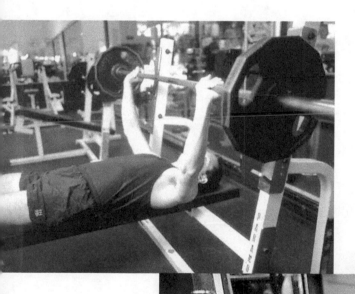

Alternative Exercise—Push-Up

Place your hands on the floor about shoulder width apart, elbows straight but not locked. Slowly lower the chest to the floor, keeping the trunk as stable as possible throughout. Push back up to the starting position and repeat.

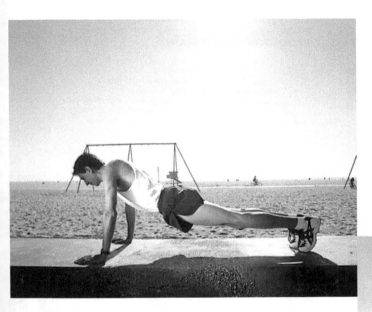

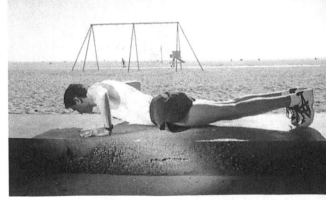

Lat Pull-Down

Sit with your knees supported by the thigh pad, feet flat on floor. Hold the bar with your hands slightly wider than shoulder width apart, palms facing forward. Keep your abs tight and lean back slightly at the hip as you pull the bar toward your chest. Pause and slowly allow your arms to return to their fully extended position. Repeat. (Avoid doing behind-the-head pull-downs, as they can cause injury.) Muscles emphasized are the latissimus dorsi, trapezius, and rhomboids.

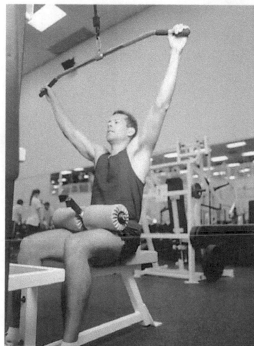

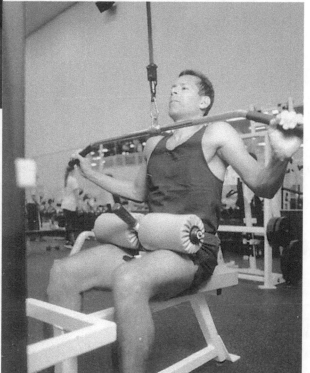

Alternative Exercise—Chin-Up

Hang fully extended from the bar with your hands slightly wider than shoulder width apart, palms facing backward. Smoothly pull up as far as you can go. Lower your body back down, maintaining full control. Muscles emphasized are the latissimus dorsi, trapezius, and rhomboid muscles.

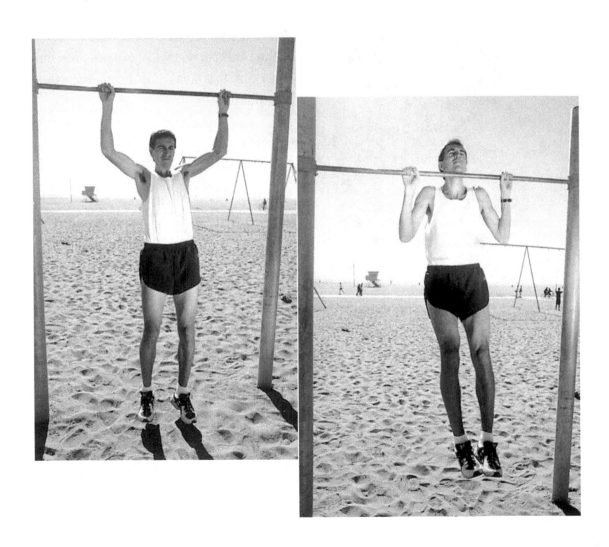

Military Press

Hold a barbell across your collarbone with palms facing forward, hands slightly wider than shoulder width apart. Your elbows should form 90-degree angles directly under the bar. Press the barbell up over your head until your arms are fully extended. Return to the starting position and repeat. Muscles emphasized are the middle deltoids and triceps.

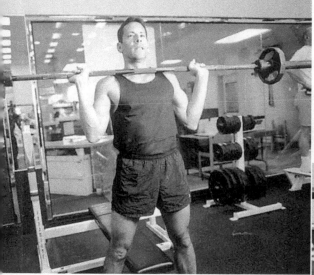

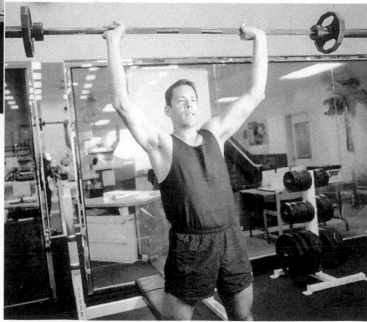

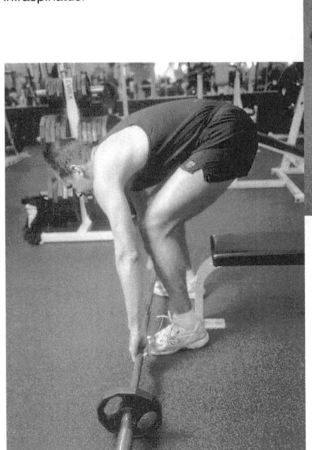

Deadlift

Bend into a squat, feet shoulder width apart, and grasp a barbell with an overhand grip, hands slightly wider than shoulder width apart. Keep your back slightly arched, your chest out, and your eyes looking forward. Slowly stand upright, keeping your arms straight and the bar close to your body. Return to the starting position and repeat. Muscles emphasized are the supraspinatus and infraspinatus.

Alternative Exercise—Superman

Lie on your stomach with your arms and legs extended. Raise your arms and legs slightly off the ground, hold for a count of 5, then lower. Repeat, trying to get your arms and legs a bit higher off the ground each time. Muscles emphasized are the supraspinatus, infraspinatus, and erector spinae.

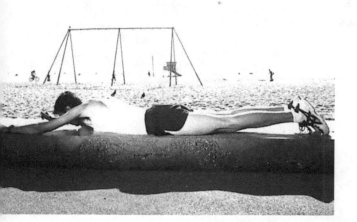

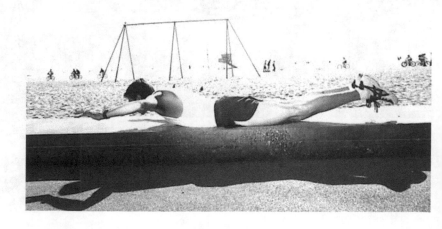

Sit-Up

Lie on floor with bent knees, feet flat on the floor, hands unclasped behind your head. Tighten the abdominals and exhale as you slowly curl up, your back neutral, just raising the shoulder blades and upper back toward the pelvis. Hold, then slowly lower and repeat. Work other abdominal muscles by curling up and rotating your left elbow towards your right knee, then right elbow to left knee, and repeat. Muscles emphasized are the rectus abdominis and external and internal obliques.

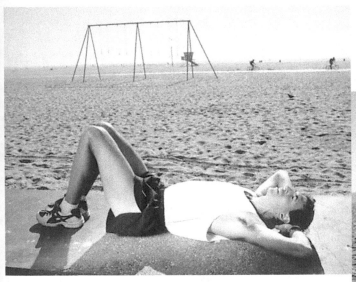

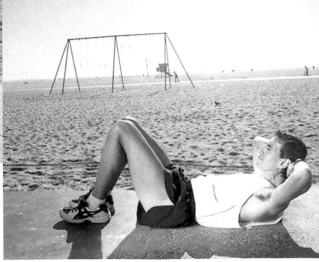

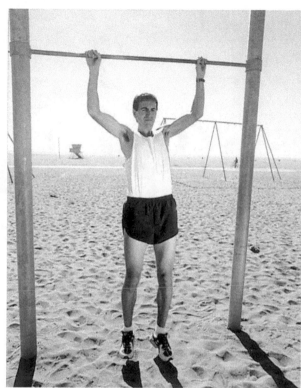

Leg Lift

Using an elevated Roman chair or pull-up bar, support yourself on your forearms with your legs dangling. Lift your knees together so that your thighs are parallel to the floor, then slowly return to the starting position and repeat. Muscles emphasized are the rectus abdominis and the external and internal obliques.

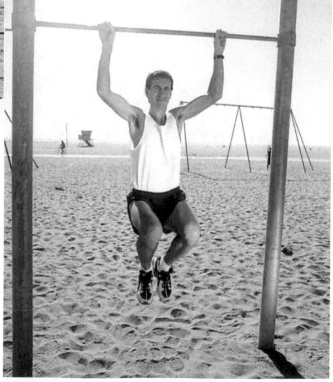

Bicep Curl

Hold a barbell or a pair of dumbbells at arm's length, palms turned so that your wrists face front. Bend your elbows to raise the weights to your shoulders without moving your upper arms. Return to the starting position and repeat. Muscles emphasized are the biceps.

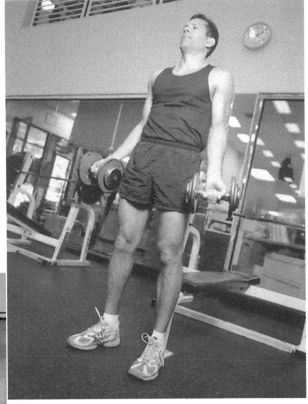

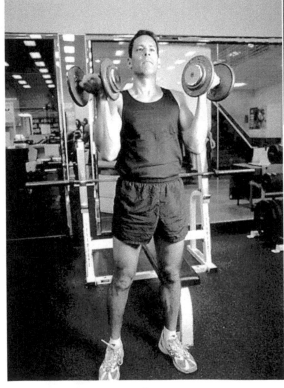

Alternative Exercise—Tricep Dip

Work the antagonist to the bicep by sitting on a chair or bench, hands gripping the front edge, legs straight out in front of you or slightly bent. Move your hips forward until they're just off the seat, then lower them slowly towards the floor. Press back up until your arms are almost fully extended, but don't lock your elbows. Muscles emphasized are the triceps.

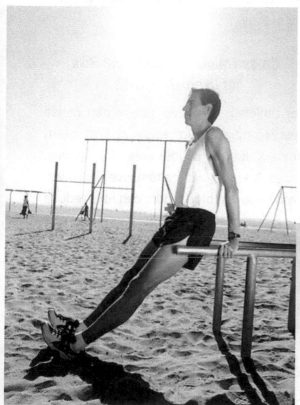

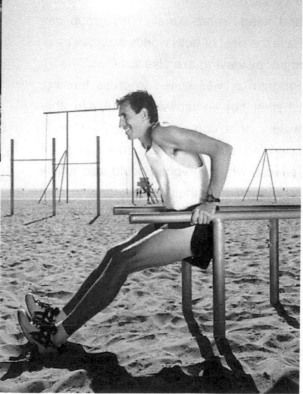

Cross Training

Many people feel comfortable doing only "their thing," be it pounding out miles on the road, swimming laps, or conquering Everest via the stair climber. Other people go crazy without variety in their workouts and ping-pong from one activity to the next. They're the ones with the garages full of athletic equipment.

There's a third group of people who are prevented by injuries, environment, or time constraints from pursuing a particular activity as often as they'd like. Or, maybe they just have a low threshold for boredom and need more variety. This group can have the best of both worlds by cross training or by varying exercise activities. The I.T. Program is well suited to cross training, whether it be an occasional dabble in other waters or a completely integrated multi-sport workout plan. In fact, there are good reasons why everyone should add a little cross training to their I.T. Program.

Cross Training Develops Different Muscles

Cross training with an exercise that is nothing like your usual activity—such as swimming for a stair climbing fanatic or cyclist—develops different, underused muscles and allows more balanced development.

Any high-intensity exercise improves the cardiovascular system, so there's no fitness advantage to always sticking to a single activity.

Cross Training Reduces the Risk of Overuse Injuries

For athletes, repetitive motion can cause overuse injuries, such as stress fractures in runners' feet or saddle sores for cyclists. Cross training with alternative activities, even once in a blue moon, can help reduce the risk of overuse injuries. It can also prevent burnout, another symptom of over-training, usually characterized by lingering aches and pains, troubled sleep, loss of appetite, weight loss, persistent colds, listlessness, sluggishness, and irritability.

Cross Training Can Be More Interesting

No doubt about it, a change now and then can be psychologically stimulating. Cross training adds interest and keeps you out of workout ruts.

Here's how to best incorporate cross training into your I.T. Program. Try one new activity once or twice a week on Active Rest Days, doing roughly two-thirds of your baseline workout. Don't do any hard workouts with this new activity until your body gets used to the new demands. Active Rest

Days are meant for recovery, so save your energy for the more intense I.T. and XL Workouts.

If you eventually want to take on a different activity for your I.T. and XL Workouts every once in a while, there's only one rule: do it hard enough so that you're tired!

This may be tricky at first, when you don't have a well-developed frame of reference and aren't sure how hard to push. If running on a treadmill is your primary I.T. Workout, for example, you know what you're capable of in terms of number of repetitions, intensity levels, and length of intervals. But in terms of mountain biking, say, your sense of your capabilities may be fuzzier. Can you really make it to the next ridge without running out of steam? It's going to take some experimenting, so just concentrate on getting in a good workout. Try doing it free-form at first: do a short warm-up, then go hard for a bit, then back off, repeating for however long you wish. Or, do it the more traditional way, going one minute at a higher intensity, followed by two minutes of active recovery. Either way, just let it rip. Charge the hill! Sprint the next lap! Boldly go to levels you've never gone to before.

If you decide to cross train on a day scheduled for a XL Workout, plan on doing it for less time and at an even lower inten-sity than you would your usual activity. If you want to continue with the new activity, slowly adjust variables over the course of several sessions until you reach an optimal I.T. and XL Workout. Keep an open mind, too—you may find you like the new cross-training activity better, and eventually switch so that it's your primary form of exercise. Continue to strike a balance between the different types of I.T. Workouts, doing longer repetitions some days and shorter ones the next, varying the number of reps, intensity level, and interval length, emphasizing both aerobic and anaerobic systems. Of course, if you don't want to push yourself hard with this new activity, just do it for fun and to break the monotony on Active Rest Days.

Stretching

It's hard to believe how much debate there's been over the years about such a simple thing as stretching. Experts argue over when it should be done, how much it should be done, and even whether it should be done at all. All things considered, stretching—if done correctly—can be highly beneficial. And yet there are many of us who still think of stretching as we think of flossing—a necessary evil, something that's good for us but has to be endured.

Many athletes skip the stretching portion of their workout entirely, opting instead to cram in an extra repetition or 2. But a better plan would be skip those last few reps and devote some quality minutes to improving flexibility instead.

It's a proven fact that the range of motion of joints decreases with age, as muscles, tendons, and ligaments grow stiffer and lose elasticity. This, coupled with the fact that muscles tend to tighten and shorten with greater use, means that loss of flexibility is inevitable unless you put up a determined fight against it. Many athletes learn this the hard way. There are any number of runners out there, for example, who find it impossible to touch their toes! You can spot them at the side of the track, hunching in vain over their stiff-as-a-board hamstrings.

Why is flexibility such a big deal? For one thing, good flexibility is a factor in staying injury-free. No one really can say just why this is, but there seems to be a connection between lack of flexibility and exercise-induced muscle damage (micro tears, not acute strains or sprains). A regular program of stretching not only can restore lost flexibility, but it also helps prevent further losses, reduces post-exercise soreness, and soothes stressed-out minds. And exercise just feels better

when the body is limber and in sync all over. Tight neck and shoulder muscles, for example, can affect form just as much as tight hamstrings. In short, stretching is time well spent. Here are a few tips for making it part of your daily routine:

Don't Stretch Cold Muscles and Joints

It's enough to make us cringe sometimes, remembering how people once advised thorough stretching before warming up. Yikes. Stretching cold muscles and joints is one sure way to do serious damage. You can avoid this by warming up a bit first, doing a few minutes of light exercise, doing your stretches, and then starting the more intense part of your workout. Or, stretch afterwards, as many people seem to prefer. Sometimes, the best part of a hard workout is the leisurely stretch that follows it.

Stretch Gently

Stretch often, and stretch gently. Too many exercisers just grab a leg and yank it back for a mere second or 2 or, even worse, stretch by bouncing. Other people stretch too long—a stretch really shouldn't be held more than 30 seconds or so. Scary fact: once a connective tissue (a ligament or tendon) is overstretched, it never returns to its normal length, and the joint associated with it will always be less stable. Don't try to pull yourself into dramatically deeper stretches. These simply activate the stretch reflex, causing the muscle to contract as self-protection against possible injury. Keep it gentle, brief, and as smooth and steady as possible.

Stretching Shouldn't Be Painful

You should feel tension when you stretch, but no pain. If it hurts, you're overdoing it and should back off, immediately. Slowly exhale and lean into the stretch just until you feel mild discomfort, then ease off a bit and hold for about 30 seconds.

Good Form Is Key

It's absurdly easy to be lazy and "cheat" when stretching, which can cause more harm than doing no stretching at all. Maintain good form by keeping the number of stretches you do down to a minimum, so you can really concentrate on what you're doing.

Do 1 Minute of Stretching for Every 10 Minutes of Exercise

Some athletes figure that 2 minutes of fast, sloppy stretches after a workout means they've stretched. It doesn't. A good rule of thumb is to do 1 minute of stretching for every 10 minutes of exercise. Allow enough time after each and every workout for a full body session, working—at the very least—the calves, hamstrings, quadriceps, lower back, shoulders, and neck.

Be Patient

Improving flexibility is no different from trying to get stronger or faster; it takes time and practice. Be patient and do it consistently, and you'll see improvements in your range of motion.

Quadriceps Stretch

Hold your ankle in one hand and gently pull your heel towards your rear end. Hold onto a wall or chair if necessary to maintain balance. Flex the foot to increase the stretch along the front of the thigh. Don't let your bent leg drift out to the side, which puts stress on the knee. Keep your hips tucked under, your back straight, and try not to lean forward.

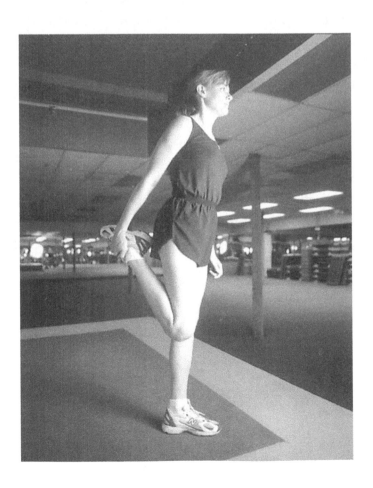

Hamstring Stretch

Prop up your leg at knee height (not hip height) or even lower to reduce the risk of injury. Bend your knee slightly and gently lean forward, keeping your back straight. You can also lie on your back, with one leg bent with the foot on the floor and the other leg upright. Pull the upright leg towards your chest with the knee slightly bent.

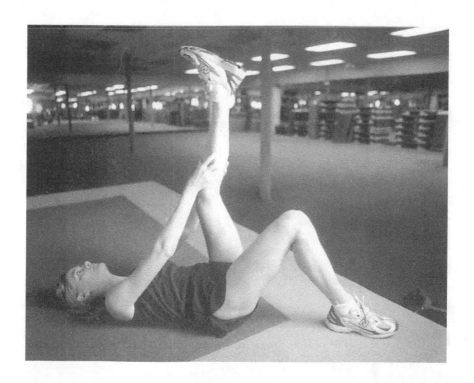

Hip Flexor Stretch

Lunge forward with your right foot, knee bent at a 90-degree angle directly over the ankle, left leg extended behind you. Lean your chest forward and let your hips sink toward the floor. Another good move: lie on your back, knees bent, feet flat on the floor. Cross the left ankle in front of the right knee. Clasp your hands behind the right knee and gently pull it towards your chest, using it as a lever to stretch the left hip. Be careful to keep the right leg bent and hold for about 30 seconds.

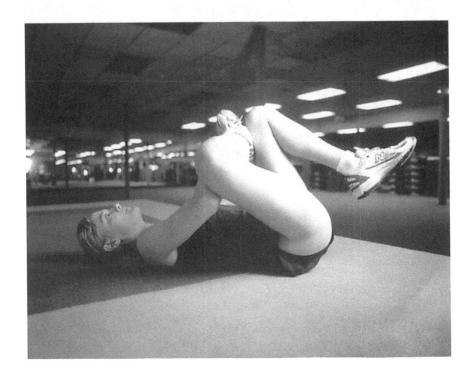

Calf Stretch

The popular way to do this stretch is to hang the heels off a step, which can tear muscles and tendons. A better method is to prop your toes against a wall, step, or tree with the heel on the ground. You can also plant both feet on the ground and lean forward, pushing against a wall or other surface.

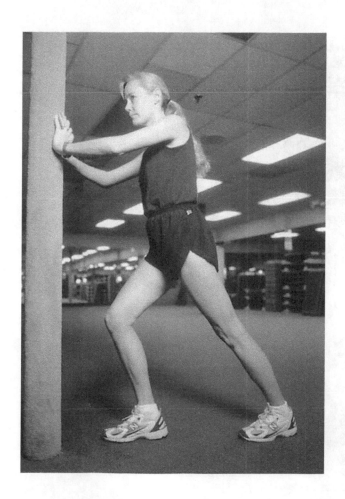

Neck and Shoulder Stretch

This is a good stretch to relieve tension and tightness in the neck and shoulders, especially for runners who let their shoulders drift towards their ears at faster paces and cyclists who hunch over their handlebars too long. Sit with a straight back, tip your head towards your chest, and hold. You may lightly touch the back of your head to enhance the stretch a bit. Do the same from side to side, gently tilting your ear towards your shoulder. You can also lie on your back, tucking your chin towards your chest while flexing your feet. Hold for a few seconds, then relax and release all tension. Try it in bed at night just before going to sleep.

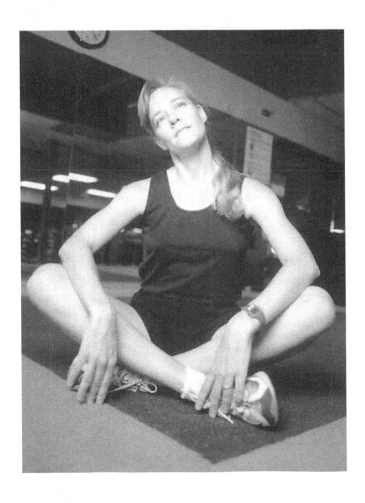

Figure-4 Stretch

Sit on the floor with one leg extended in front of you, toes pointed up. Bend the other leg so the sole of the foot rests against the opposite thigh just below your groin (making a "4"). Lean forward, reaching for your toes with both arms, and exhale while keeping a straight back until you feel the stretch.

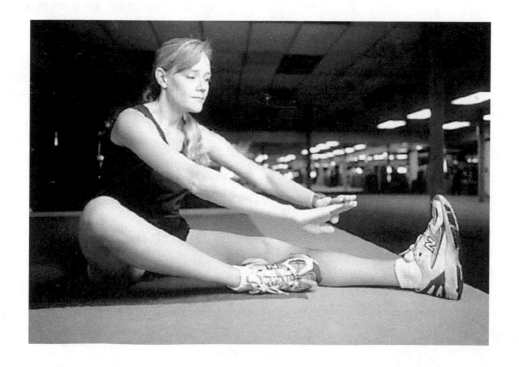

Injury Prevention

Athletes and injuries seem to go together, usually because we do too much, too fast, with too little time set aside for rest and recovery. There are many ways to avoid injury, however, and quick action to counter minor problems can keep them from turning into chronic ones.

The single best way to prevent injury is to avoid overtraining. Cross train and strength train to help develop other muscle groups and provide balance and rest for your primary movers. Watch for early signs of burnout. And, learn to recognize differences in pain.

Good Pain vs. Harmful Pain

"Good pain" is common, exercise-induced muscle soreness and is often relieved by a warm-up. "Harmful pain" is not relieved by a warm-up or rest and indicates a genuine injury. Some other fine-line distinctions between the two are as follows:

- Muscle soreness is mildly uncomfortable and disappears rapidly. An injury usually feels more acute, like a sharp jolt of electricity or a pop, and lasts longer. (Exceptions are overuse injuries, which tend to have a more gradual onset.)

- Overuse injuries (such as stress fractures) come about from the wear and tear of repetitive movement, such as running and cycling. These injuries may have no obvious cause and often don't seem like a big deal at first—they're just a dull, annoying pain. But these injuries are actually hairline fractures in bone or microtears in muscle and, if ignored, can turn into bigger problems.

- Muscle soreness tends to be on both sides of the body, while injury is usually one-sided.

- Injury tends to be more point specific ("It hurts here"), while muscle soreness is more diffuse.

- Soreness usually goes away after a day or 2. It responds well to R.I.C.E. (rest, ice, compression, and elevation) and anti-inflammatories, such as ibuprofen. Pain associated with an injury lingers longer.

Tips to Avoid Injury

When You Feel Pain, Stop Immediately

Stop immediately whenever you feel pain. Oftentimes, you don't feel any pain until the damage is already done, so you'll just make things worse by struggling to work through it.

Slowly Increase Training Intensity over Time

Don't fall into the trap of doing too much, too soon. Increase each variable one at a time and listen to your body.

Limit Hard Training to 4- to 8-Week Periods

Limit hard training to 4- to 8-week periods, then ease off to give your body a breather. You can't continually increase training intensity without a break—push hard enough, long enough, and your body will eventually come to a screeching halt. Maintain control over your workout program by factoring in recovery periods before your body reaches the breaking point. Elite athletes are no exception.

Use Good Form and Technique

Sacrificing good form and technique in order to finish a tough workout session means you're not fully in control of your body—and that's when injuries happen.

Don't Skimp on Active Rest Days

Surprisingly, light exercise can promote healing faster than fanning yourself on the veranda all day. So don't skimp on Active Rest Days—get moving!

Try Cross Training while Recovering from Injury

Don't use injury as an excuse to become a complete slug (unless it's severe, of course). Instead, try cross training while you recover. Do what's pain free—if you have shin splints, try swimming. Shoulder problems? Get on a bike instead or "run" in a pool to avoid heavy pounding, as many competitive athletes often do. Cross training will keep you fit and also prevent the muscle imbalances and inflexibility that come from doing only a single sport.

What to do if you're feeling pain? Take a few days off with R.I.C.E., the basic first aid for any sport-related injury.

Rest

Rest, by backing off completely for a few days, or find a light, nonaggravating exercise to do until you fully recover.

Ice

Apply ice, a cold pack, or a bag of frozen veggies for 10 to 15 minutes every 2 to 4 hours to relieve pain and reduce any swelling. (If the swelling is down after 48 hours of ice treatments, do a little heat treatment to speed up the healing process, using heat pads, moist hot packs, hot baths, or a soak in a whirlpool.)

Compression

Put on an elastic wrap, with firm but comfortable pressure, during and after an ice treatment. Make sure you take it off before sleeping.

Elevation

Prop up the injured area so it's elevated above heart level whenever possible.

You might take some aspirin, ibuprofen, or naproxen to reduce pain and swelling, too, but read the dosage information carefully and don't start popping them like candy (as too many athletes tend to do). You shouldn't have to take a pain reliever to get through a workout! And, don't make the mistake of trying to exercise "through the pain," especially if there's any chance you have more acute tissue dam-age. Some world-class athletes do this and seem to bounce right back after injury—but they have ex-perts to diagnose and treat them immediately, they're in tip-top condition, and they're highly motivated to recover. Stop exercising whenever there's pain beyond mild discomfort, and rest to avoid aggravating the problem. If there's no improvement or the pain gets worse, get thee to an orthopedist, a specialist in musculoskeletal and joint problems.

There's no question that you're going to experience some muscle soreness doing the I.T. Program. The greater intensity leaves most people "feeling it" the next day or two after a hard workout. But continued soreness should be countered by skipping the next I.T. or XL Workout and taking 1 to 3 days off. Resume exercise with a few Active Rest Days once you're pain-free again, then go back to I.T. and XL Workouts at a slightly lower intensity for a few sessions. And don't worry about losing speed or endurance when taking time off to recover from injury—you won't lose fitness as quickly as you might think. Keep the big picture in mind. An injury is a minor setback when caught early enough, and time on the couch can keep it from becoming serious enough to really interfere with your workout schedule.

Your Notes:

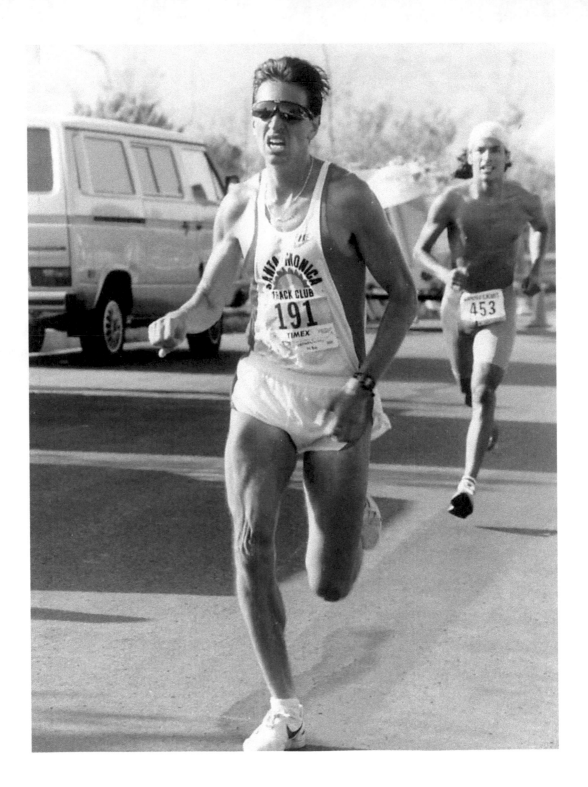

The I.T. Competitive Edge Program

The roar of the crowd is deafening as you surge from the pack on the way to certain victory. The finish line comes into view, your outstretched arms wave to the screaming crowd, and...

You wake up.

Okay, so most of us compete better in our dreams than in reality. But that doesn't mean it's impossible to set personal records and feel the same pride as guys with gold medals around their necks. The I.T. Program works because it employs the same basic training methods used by elite athletes, and the principles of physiologic adaptation are the same for everyone from Olympic champions to weekend warriors in hometown 5Ks.

The rigors of athletic competition aren't for everyone. Some people want nothing at all to do with it. They exercise strictly for fitness or fun or a sense of well-being, and if they do enter a race, it's to raise money for a good cause or it's a chance to wear a crazy team costume with the gang from the office. And, that's fine. But these folks might want to skip the rest of this chapter, which is written for those who think the whole point of exercise is to push their limitations, a chance to get out there and see what the ol' bod can do. When a good race rolls around, they sign up, go the distance, and head home wearing a new T-shirt and a smug, satisfied smile. Or—as it often happens—they wonder if they could have done better and how they might improve their results next time.

Performing at peak level requires a master plan, a carefully choreographed mix of workouts designed to get the most out of your body—the I.T. Competitive Edge Program. This training schedule is even more challenging than the standard I.T. Program and requires discipline and a strong drive to go faster than ever before. Accepting the challenge—and the fatigue and aching muscles that invariably go along with it—can bring you closer to fulfilling your true physical potential than you may have believed possible.

Choose a Challenge

First things first: select a specific challenge for yourself, something to genuinely test your capabilities. The key word here is "specific." Instead of a wishy-washy vow to "run faster," say "I want to run a 5K in under 17 minutes" or "I want to bike from here to Tallahassee in 2 hours." As in so many other aspects of life, having a specific destination is the only way to ever get anywhere.

This challenge can be done as a time trial or as part of an organized competition. A time trial is a full-effort exertion done over a particular distance, such as a 1-mile swim, and it's just you racing against the clock. Time trials are a good way to track progress, but they have one significant drawback: you cannot replicate the feel of a race in training, no matter how intensely you work out. That's why personal bests—and world records—are rarely (if ever) recorded alone, even by the most talented, motivated athlete. Because of this, we'll stick to discussing organized competitions, such as foot races or open swims or cycling criteriums, in which the adrenaline rush of going head-to-head with other athletes can lead to faster times than you might reach on your own.

Timing Is Everything

Successful competitors know that timing is everything. Find a race that's at least 4 months away, preferably 6. Attaining peak fitness involves much more than a quick pre-race tune-up—you need enough time to give your training a real overhaul. Elite athletes often train for 6 months to a year before peaking within a 4- to 6-week competitive window of opportunity. Then, after a period of much-needed rest and recovery, they start the process all over again. To succeed, you need that same discipline and dedication to gut through the tough times, those dark days when you're tired or

Pushing the Envelope: The Anaerobic Threshold

The I.T. Program prepares you for the rigors of competition by increasing the body's anaerobic threshold, or AT. As long as there's enough oxygen in a working muscle, and the muscle is able to use that oxygen, exercise is considered aerobic and can keep going for quite some time. As intensity increases, the body's ability to deliver and utilize oxygen to generate energy is overwhelmed, so energy has to be created anaerobically. Breathing is labored and the heart rate is cranked up nearly to its maximum at this point. Anaerobic metabolism results in the secretion of lactic acid into the blood, where the liver and heart tap it as an energy source. Above a certain exercise intensity, more of this waste product is produced than can be processed (or cleared) by the body, and it starts to build up in the blood. This level of exercise is known as the "anaerobic threshold,"

where the increased amount of lactic acid limits how long the body can continue exercising at a high intensity. And that's what hampers performance during workouts and competition.

The I.T. Program helps battle this barrier by training the body to work at higher intensities for longer periods of time before reaching the anaerobic threshold. Long endurance-type workouts, such as XL Workouts, delay anaerobic exercise by creating more muscle capillaries and mitochondria to use oxygen more efficiently. Regular I.T. Workouts and AT (Anaerobic Threshold) Workouts also buff up the rate of lactate clearance and retrain some larger muscle fibers to make better use of oxygen. The net result of all these physical adaptations is the ability to better manage the hard work of a grueling workout or athletic competition, both physically and psychologically.

the water's freezing or it's pouring rain and the race seems a million years away. But for anyone with a spark of competitive instinct, this is what training is all about. If it were easy, everyone would be doing it, right?

Take Small, Progressive Steps

Plan to do some practice races or individual time trials as your target competition approaches. It's a great way to stay motivated and gives you a good sense of your physical condition. With each race or time trial, your goal is to gain racing experience and progressively lower your times. These smaller, progressive steps are important; no one, no matter how naturally gifted they are, wakes up one morning, decides to take up running, and manages to qualify for the Olympics by dinnertime. Choose these short-term goals carefully; completing short, fast races as well as longer, endurance-oriented competitions builds speed, stamina, and a sense of pace. Be sure to allow yourself enough time to both train and recover—use this chapter to figure out when to schedule these practice races so they don't end up hindering your ultimate goal.

Periodization

It sounds like a dental procedure, but "periodization" simply means breaking your training into distinct blocks of time to focus on developing particular physiologic systems. Many elite athletes divide their training time into four basic phases:

1. Endurance (aerobic) phase

2. Stamina (aerobic/anaerobic) phase

3. Speed (anaerobic) phase

4. Rest/Competition phase

The idea is to start off training "long and slow" and gradually work toward "short and fast," strengthening both aerobic and anaerobic systems along the way. Done correctly, this brings you to the threshold of peak performance just prior to your target race. If there's any secret behind world-class athletic performance, this might very well be it.

Time to get to work.

Count the number of weeks between today and the date of the race, then organize that time into four phases: Endurance, Stamina, Speed, and Rest/Competition. Allow 2 to 4 weeks for the last phase, and divide the other three phases into equal blocks of time. For example, if the race is in 16 weeks, allow about 4 weeks each for Phases One through Three, and 4 weeks for the Rest/Competition phase. For a 6-month cycle, or 26 weeks, allow 8 weeks each for the first three phases, 2 weeks for the last. Add any leftover days to the Endurance phase.

Next, plan a workout schedule for each phase according to whether you need to concentrate on speed (for races under 30 minutes) or endurance (for races longer than 30 minutes). Then all that's left is to follow through with the plan and just do it.

Short-Distance I.T. vs. Long-Distance I.T.

The I.T. Peak Performance Program has two concentrations:

Short-Distance I.T.

Long-Distance I.T.

Select either one of these to concentrate on during each phase, depending on the length of your chosen race. Short-Distance I.T. is designed to prepare you for competitions under 30 minutes; Long-

Distance I.T. is geared for events lasting 30 minutes plus. Within these two divisions are various small adjustments that can be made to tailor your workouts even further. For the purposes of specific workouts, we'll assume that your baseline workout time is about 50 minutes (plus another 10 for stretching). If your actual workout time is substantially less or more than this, adjust the following workouts accordingly.

Some abbreviations used in this chapter are as follows:

WU =   warm-up (to be done at an easy pace)

CD =   cooldown (also done at an easy pace)

I.T. =   Interval Training Workout

XL =   Extra Long Workout

AT =   Aerobic Threshold Workout

AR =   Active Rest Day

min =   minute(s)

sec =   second(s)

What If I Miss Workouts Because I'm Too Busy, Ill, or Injured?

If you have to miss a workout because of a genuine lack of time, try to miss an Active Rest Day. These are mainly designed to be recovery days anyway, so not much will be lost. Missing an occasional "hard" workout (I.T., AT, or XL) is fine too—your fitness level won't go to pot if you skip a session here or there. If you need to miss a number of days because you're sick or injured, by all means do so. When you're ready, start back up again gradually with a few Active Rest Days before moving on to the more intense workouts (the first few of these should be scaled back a bit, too). If you're missing workouts because of a lack of motivation, be honest with yourself and reassess your goals, then adjust your schedule accordingly. You don't have to do a workout just because it's on the schedule!

Phase One: Endurance Training

The physiologic goal of this endurance-training phase is to develop more extensive capillary beds and mitochondria so that working muscles are able to use more oxygen (this is known as "aerobic metabolism"). You build endurance as your body develops natural coping mechanisms in response to the stress, learning to better hoard fuel and fluid, to parcel out energy so that it lasts as long as possible, and to reduce wasted motion so every stride or stroke is ultraefficient. Just as important as these physical adaptations are the psychological ones. Putting in the time when your target race is still a good ways off helps toughen up mental resolve and hones discipline and willpower, which you definitely need to succeed. For this reason, Phase One includes 2 XL Workouts and 1 I.T. Workout a week to concentrate on developing aerobic metabolism. Don't be disappointed if you don't improve every single week—nobody does. The human body goes through cycles, so be prepared to have bad patches during which you can't accomplish as much as before. Be patient and you'll eventually see gains.

Here's how Phase One looks if you are focusing on short distances:

Phase One: Short-Distance I.T. Program/XL Workouts

The first of your 2 weekly XL Workouts does not actually involve going long at all. Instead, focus on going slightly harder than your baseline aerobic workout, keeping the intensity constant for the whole workout. Finish feeling tired but able to go a bit longer (say, 25 percent more) if you had to. Over the course of this phase, gradually increase intensity, but be careful not to get too gung ho and push yourself at race pace yet. At this point, you're just letting your body adjust to moderately faster paces sustained for longer periods of time.

For your second weekly XL Workout, gradually increase your workout time to 75 minutes (or 50 percent longer than your baseline aerobic workout) by the final 2 weeks of this phase. This extended time/distance may seem like a rather substantial leap within a relatively short period. Just keep the intensity low-to-moderate and you should stay right on track.

Phase One: Short-Distance I.T. Program/I.T. Workouts

Do a single session of interval training each week, with 1-minute repetitions and 2-minute intervals. Use the first few workouts to find the right intensity, then gradually increase the number of repetitions until you're doing about 50 percent more by the end of the phase. Don't mess with the repetition length or the interval length. Let your body guide each workout and don't push to do more if it isn't ready. Strive to finish each workout tired but able to continue on a bit longer if necessary.

Here's a breakdown of the Phase One: Short-Distance I.T. Program.

Day 1:   XL
WU 5 min
35 min of continuous faster-paced activity, with increasing intensity over course of phase
CD 5 min

Day 2:   AR (25–35 minutes at slow pace)

Day 3:   I.T.
WU 10–15 min
8 x 1-min reps/2-min rest, increasing to 12 reps by end of phase
CD 5–10 min

Day 4:   Day off

Day 5: XL (start at 60 min and build to 75 min at a modest pace by end of phase)

Day 6: AR

Day 7: AR

Note: Active Rest Days do not change throughout the I.T. Competitive Edge Program

Here's what to do for Phase One if you're focusing on long distances:

Phase One: Long-Distance I.T. Program/XL Workouts

Do 2 XL Workouts a week during this phase. The first workout is the shorter one. In addition to a short warm-up and cooldown, do up to 45 minutes of continuous exercise (for races 30–60 minutes long) or up to 1 hour (for longer races) at your baseline aerobic workout level of effort. Once you work up to the maximum time, gradually start upping the intensity. Use a workout log to track how you feel from day to day, and adjust your workouts accordingly.

The second workout depends on the length of your target race. Let's say it's a 10K run, which you figure will take more than 30 minutes and less than an hour. With this in mind, you need to gradually increase the duration of your workout until it's 90 minutes long. For events longer than an hour, such as a half marathon or a long bike race, build up to 2 hours. (Events longer than 2 hours will be dealt with later in this chapter.) Do these workouts at a modest pace, focusing on just completing the distance.

Note: Don't increase training time by more than 20 percent in a single week.

Too much additional training time is just asking for burnout or an overuse injury. Aim for the sought-after "tired but could keep going" feeling, adjusting your time and pace accordingly. If you can't manage to complete a full XL Workout at least once during this phase, pick another race so there's extra time to prepare, or spend more time on this phase and shorten Phase Two and Phase Three.

Phase One: Long-Distance I.T. Program/I.T. Workout

Do interval training once a week, using 1-minute reps and 2-minute intervals. Spend the first few workouts finding the right intensity level, then focus on increasing the number of reps by about 50 percent over the course of this phase. Stick with the same interval and repetition length—the emphasis here is on getting used to doing a longer workout. Things will get more intense later.

Here's how a Long-Distance I.T. Program week looks for Phase One:

Day 1: XL
WU 5 min
build from 40 to 45 or 60 min,
depending on goal, with
gradual increase in
intensity over phase
CD 5 min

Day 2: AR (25–35 min at a slow pace)

Day 3: I.T.
WU 10–15 min
8 x 1-min reps/2-min
intervals, increasing number of
repetitions to 12 by end of
phase
CD 5–10 min

Day 4: Day off

Day 5: XL (build up to 90 min or 2
hours, depending on
competition goal moderate
effort)

Day 6: AR

Day 7: AR

Note: Active Rest Days do not
change throughout the I.T.
Competitive Edge Program

The last 4 to 7 days of Phase One for both short-distance and long-distance I.T.

concentrations should be strictly limited to Active Rest Days, so your body can take a breather and absorb the additional stresses being put on it. You'll be itching for action by the end of this recovery week, so try testing yourself with a time trial or a practice race, something a bit shorter or longer than the distance of your target race. If your goal is to run a 10K, for example, test yourself with either a 5K, a 5-mile, or a 15K race. For psychological reasons, try to avoid competing at your target race distance. At this early point in your training, your performance may fall well short of your expectations, which can be discouraging. Competing at alternate distances also provides some variety you might not otherwise have. Joseph typically runs three or four 5K or 10K races to prepare for an 8-mile target race every year in Honolulu. These shorter races are ideal preparation because he can run at faster tempos, yet recover more quickly than he would doing a 15K or half-marathon. No matter what race you ultimately decide to do, take whatever positive things you can from the experience and use them to keep yourself on course towards a future peak performance. Take 3 or 4 Active Rest Days or full days off after this race or time trial before starting Phase Two.

Phase Two: Stamina Training

This stamina-building phase is unique in that it develops both anaerobic and aerobic systems as the body trains to perform at high intensities for extended periods of time. This type of training is similar to the experience of actual competition, geared to teach the body to better tolerate lactic acid and fatigue.

Phase Two: Short-Distance I.T. Program/XL Workouts

Do one XL Workout a week that's 75 minutes long, or 50 percent longer than your baseline aerobic workout. This maintains a stable aerobic foundation while you work to improve stamina. If you're up to it, you can crank up the intensity a notch, but the most important thing is to just put in the time and complete the entire workout, especially since the I.T. and AT Workouts during this phase are often challenging enough.

Phase Two: Short-Distance I.T. Program/AT Workouts

An AT (Anaerobic Threshold) Workout is scheduled only once every other week. Some athletes call these sessions "lactate threshold workouts" because they develop

tolerance of lactic acid, that waste product of anaerobic metabolism that makes your legs burn after a hard repetition. The slower it pools in your muscles, the faster you can go for longer distances...and that's what sets PRs and wins races.

An AT Workout isn't easy. It's the closest thing to actual racing you'll experience in training. Here's how it works: after a 10- to 15-minute easy warm-up, do 15 minutes at a constant, high intensity, enough so that you're short of breath and unable to speak in full sentences, but not full-out racing. Think of it as a 90-percent effort and finish feeling like you only have a few more minutes at that intensity left in you. You may have to pause at the end to catch your breath, just as you might do in a race; then do a 10-minute cooldown, nice and easy. Ease up whenever you start feeling overly strained and make a note to start more conservatively next time. As your fitness improves, you'll be able to increase the pace, but never go beyond the point where you feel in complete control of the workout.

Phase Two: Short-Distance I.T. Program/I.T. Workouts

There are 2 I.T. sessions a week in Phase Two. For the first, do the same number of 1-

minute repetitions at the same pace as at the end of Phase One, but now decrease the length of each interval. For example, if your interval was 2 minutes long, slowly chop it down—to 1:45, 1:30, 1:15—stopping when you get down to 1 minute. This may sound like no big deal, but this shorter recovery time makes doing the reps at the same level of intensity a true challenge. If you're really struggling, ease off and take slightly longer intervals. By the end of this phase, you want to be doing 1-minute reps with 1-minute intervals at the same or a slightly higher level of intensity. Feel tired? Good. You're doing it right.

The second I.T. Workout of the week is done on weeks when you don't do an AT Workout. Do 5 high-intensity, 3-minute-long repetitions with 3-minute intervals (we call these "3-minute drills"). Try to keep the intensity level consistent for all the reps throughout the workout and finish feeling as if you could do 1 more rep at the same pace if you had to. After finding an intensity level that feels right for you, try to increase it gradually over the course of the phase.

Three minutes of pushing yourself hard is going to seem like an eternity at first. It's long enough to generate a significant amount of lactic acid, but brief enough so that your body can deal with it. These drills will help get you "racing fit," ready to handle the challenge of the hard, continuous effort of competition.

Note: Because of the greater level of effort required for this phase, you may need an additional day off occasionally.

Here's how the Phase Two: Short-Distance I.T. Program week breaks down:

Day 1:   AT
            WU 10–15 min
            15 min continuous high-intensity
                effort, intensity increasing
                over course of phase
            CD 5–10 min

Alternate week:

Day 1:   3-minute drills
            WU 10–15 min
            5 x 3-min reps/3-min
                intervals, intensity increasing
                over course of phase
            CD 5–10 min

Day 2:   AR or day off

Day 3:   I.T.
            WU 10–15 min
            1-min reps with
                intervals decreasing from 2-min
                to 1-min over course of phase,
                same number of reps as end of
                Phase One
            CD 5–10 min

Day 4:   AR or day off

Day 5:   XL (75 min or 50 percent longer than baseline aerobic workout, okay to up intensity level)

Day 6:   AR

Day 7:   AR

If you're focusing on longer distances, here's how to do Phase Two:

Phase Two: Long-Distance I.T. Program/XL Workouts

To train for a competition lasting 30 to 60 minutes, do a 90-minute XL Workout at a moderate level of effort once a week. For longer races, train with alternating workouts: a 90-minute session 1 week, a 2-hour session the next.

Phase Two: Long-Distance I.T. Program/AT Workouts

Do this workout every other week. It consists of 20 minutes at a constant, high intensity, enough so that you are short of breath but not full-out racing. Push yourself in a controlled manner and finish feeling like you could keep going another 3 or 4 minutes at the same intensity if you had to.

Phase Two: Long-Distance I.T. Program/I.T. Workouts

For your first of 2 weekly I.T. sessions, do the same number of 1-minute reps at the same intensity as at the end of Phase One, but decrease the length of each interval. Slowly chop it from 2 minutes down to 1:45, then 1:30, then 1:15, stopping when you get down to 1 minute.

For the second I.T. Workout (on weeks when you don't do the AT Workout), do 5-minute drills: 5 repetitions, each lasting 5 minutes, with 3-minute intervals. These longer reps are tough, but they're excellent training for longer races. Slowly increase the repetition intensity over the course of this phase, always finishing feeling as if you could do 1 or 2 more repetitions.

Here's how the Phase Two: Long-Distance I.T. Program week shapes up:

Day 1:   AT
WU 10–15 min
20-min of high-intensity effort, increasing intensity as phase progresses
CD 5–10 min

Alternate Week:

Day 1:   WU 10–15 min
5-minute drills (5 x 5-min reps/ 3-min intervals)
CD 5–10 min

Day 2:   AR or day off

Day 3:   I.T.
WU 10–15 min
12–15 1-min repetitions,
gradually decreasing interval
from 2-min down to 1-min,
same intensity and number of
reps as end of Phase One
CD 5–10 min

Day 4:   AR or day off

Day 5:   XL (90-min at moderate pace
if preparing for 30–60-min race
for longer races, alternate 90-
min sessions one week with 2-
hour session the next)

Day 6:   AR

Day 7:   AR

Allow 4 to 7 Active Rest Days at the end of this phase. If you're curious to see where you're at in terms of conditioning, sign up for a practice race or do a time trial on your own at a shorter distance than your target race. Take 3 or 4 Active Rest Days or days off after this race or time trial before beginning Phase Three.

Phase Three: Speed (Anaerobic) Phase

This phase hones you from "racing fit" to "racing sharp," using larger muscle fibers, improving efficiency, and focusing on intensities higher than that of an actual race. The end result: greater ease performing at faster speeds. Better conditioning means less struggle in the early portion of the race, so there's more reserve to kick it into another gear as the finish line approaches.

Phase Three: Short-Distance I.T. Program/XL Workouts

Every other week, go 75 minutes or 50 percent longer than your baseline aerobic workout, whichever is greater (alternate this session with the AT Workout).

Phase Three: Short-Distance I.T. Program/AT Workouts

Do 15 minutes of continuous high-intensity work at an increasing level of effort over the course of the phase (alternate this session with the XL Workout).

Phase Three: Short-Distance I.T. Program/I.T. Workouts

Do the first I.T. session of the week with 1-minute repetitions and 1-minute intervals.

But here's a new twist: to wring more intensity out of this workout, break the reps up into 4 sets (for example, divide 12 reps into 4 sets of 3 repetitions each), rounding off uneven numbers. For each set, do the first 2 reps at about the same pace as at the end of Phase Two. Crank it up a notch for the 3rd rep, staying just short of going full tilt. Increase the intensity for all repetitions accordingly over the course of this phase. Keep the same 1-minute rest period between reps and 3 easy minutes between sets.

The 2nd I.T. Workout of the week will include either:

Twelve repetitions of 30 seconds, with 1-minute intervals, or

Five repetitions lasting 2 minutes, with 3-minute intervals.

Aim to do a mix of both workouts during this training period. To prepare for shorter races, emphasize the 30-second reps, or do the longer reps to get ready for longer races. Finish every workout with that "I could keep going" feeling, tired but not completely exhausted. Again, increase repetition intensity over the course of this phase.

Here's the Phase Three: Short-Distance I.T. Program week at a glance:

Day 1:   I.T.
WU 10–15 min
3 or 4 x 1-min reps/1-min intervals, with 3-min between sets, final rep in each set done at even greater intensity
CD 5–10 min

Day 2:   AR

Day 3:   I.T.
WU 10–15 min
12 x 30-sec reps/1-min intervals, or 5 x 2-min reps/3-min intervals, depending on target race length
CD 5–10 min

Day 4:   Day off

Day 5:   XL (75-min or 50 percent longer than baseline workout, whichever is greater)

Alternate week:

Day 5:   AT
WU 10–15 min
15-min of high-intensity effort
CD 5–10 min

Day 6:   AR or day off

Day 7:   AR

Here's how to do Phase Three if you're concentrating on longer distances:

Phase Three: Long-Distance I.T. Program/XL Workouts

This once-a-week session should last about 90 minutes, at a moderate pace, if you're training for competitions of 30–60 minutes. For longer races, alternate 90-minute sessions with 2-hour sessions.

Phase Three: Endurance I.T. Program/I.T. Workouts

Do the first I.T. session of the week with 1-minute repetitions and 1-minute intervals. But, to make things even more intense, break the reps up into 4 sets (for example, divide 12 reps into 4 sets of 3), rounding off uneven numbers. For each set, do the first 2 reps at about the same pace as at the end of Phase Two. Increase the effort level for the 3rd rep, staying just short of maximum speed. Do 3 easy minutes between sets. Remember to increase the intensity over the course of the phase.

For your 2nd I.T. Workout of the week, you have a choice of 2 workouts:

Five sets of 2-minute reps with 3-minute intervals, or

Five sets of 5-minute reps with 3-minute intervals.

Find an intensity level that lets you finish feeling tired but able to keep going a bit longer if necessary, then increase that ef-fort level over the course of this phase as your fitness improves.

Here's what the Phase Three: Long-Distance I.T. Program week looks like.

Day 1:   I.T.
WU 10–15 min
4 sets of 3–4 x 1-min repetitions with 1-min interval, done at same intensity as at the end of Phase Two
CD 5–10 min

Day 2:   AR

Day 3:   I.T.
WU 10–15 min
5 x 2 min reps/3-min interval; alternate this with 5 x 5-min reps/3-min intervals, with intensity increasing over phase
CD 5–10 min

Day 4:   Day off

Day 5:   XL (90-min at moderate pace if preparing for 30–60-min race, or alternate 90-min sessions with 2-hour sessions to prepare for longer races)

Day 6:   AR or day off

Day 7:   AR

You won't need to take any additional Active Rest Days at the end of Phase Three, since Phase Four emphasizes lighter training in preparation for competition.

Phase Four: Rest/ Competition Phase

The Rest and Competition phase tends to be the one that athletes screw up the most. Improved speed, stamina, and endurance should have you on the brink of realizing your physical potential, but if you're burned out from overtraining, all that hard work is completely useless. Don't sabotage things by training hard right up until race day.

If you're going to race hard, you have to race smart.

In order to give it everything you've got in competition, your body needs adequate rest before race day. Think back to the practice races or time trials you did between phases, how they came after several Active Rest Days, with another 3 or 4 easy days or full days off before you advanced to the next phase. During Phase Four, staying fresh and rested is of even greater importance.

Assuming your target race coincides with the end of Phase Four, you want to squeeze in one to three time trials or practice races during this phase before the big day arrives. Why test yourself at this stage of the game? Two reasons: it's another opportunity to practice performing at maximum effort, and it provides a chance to achieve personal bests (and a shot of confidence) at a shorter distance than your target race. Unlike in the first two phases, make sure these practice races or time trials are shorter than your target race distance, because longer races require more time for recovery. For instance, if you're planning on a 10K for your target race, practice with a 5K race or a 1-mile time trial. If possible, try to keep all practice races under 30 minutes, no matter what distance the target race is. If you want to do a longer race, do it between the earlier phases (or, better yet, save it for after you successfully complete your target race).

The mantra for Phase Four is "less is more." For the next 3 to 6 weeks, decrease the length of all your workouts by 30 to 40 percent (even Active Rest Days), while keeping your intensity level the same as in Phase Three. (Athletes call this "tapering," and studies show that it is the best way to maintain peak fitness for a window of 4 to 6 weeks). The week of your target race, chop your workouts in half. You should feel pumped up and fresh at the end of these workouts, not tired. Skip the last I.T. Workout and make sure you have at least 4 days of active rest or days off just prior to the race. This helps keep your body fresh and injury-free.

Here's how a tapering week looks for the Phase Four: Short-Distance I.T. Program:

Day 1: I.T.
WU 10–15 min
2 sets of 3–4 1-min repetitions/1-min intervals, with last rep of each set done at a slightly higher intensity
CD 5–10 min

Day 2: AR (two-thirds as long as usual)

Day 3: I.T.
WU 10–15 min
6–8 x 30-sec reps/1-min intervals, or 3 2-min reps/3-min intervals
CD 5–10 min

Note: If target race is on Day 7, substitute an Active Rest Day here.

Day 4: Day off

Day 5: AR (two-thirds as long as usual)

Day 6: AR (one-third as long as usual)

Day 7: XL (45 min at moderate pace) or target race

Here's how a tapering week looks for the Phase Four: Long-Distance I.T. Program, with a race on Day 7:

Day 1: I.T.
WU 10–15 min
2 sets of 3–4 1-min repetitions/1-min intervals, with last rep of each set done at slightly higher intensity
CD 5–10 min

Day 2: AR (two-thirds as long as usual)

Day 3: I.T.
WU 10–15 min
3 2-min reps/3-min intervals, or 3 5-min reps/3-min intervals
CD 5–10 min

Note: If target race is on Day 7, substitute an Active Rest Day here.

Day 4: Day off

Day 5: AR (two-thirds as long as usual)

Day 6: AR (one-third as long as usual)

Day 7: XL (60 min at moderate pace) or target race

What should you do with all the extra pent-up energy you no doubt have? Simple. Relax and store it up! You're going to need it on race day.

Don't succumb to the temptation to dabble in other physical activities or fill your day with chores or make any drastic changes in your routine right before a big race. Remember, you're not training to train, you're training to race. Take things easy to conserve as much energy as possible and be a sloth for a few days—you'll more than make up for it when it comes time to compete. At this point, psychological preparation is just as important as your physical training, so spend your time on the sofa even more productively by doing some mind exercises known as "visualization."

Visualization:
The Mental Edge Revisited

The only way to perform at a maximum level is to have a clear mental picture of what you plan to do before you do it. Elite athletes use this sort of visualization all the time. Positive visualization—as well as negative visualization—provides the mental edge necessary to reach your physical peak.

Positive visualization is basically a detailed daydream about your upcoming competition that plays over and over inside your head. Say you're getting ready for a big 10K. Visualize the race from start to finish: standing on the line, the start gun firing, your legs striding through the early stages, feeling completely in control, pacing yourself well. Picture the midpoint of the race, when you're beginning to feel tired from the effort but able to push hard through the fatigue. Picture moving with strength and confidence, maintaining good form as you move up through the field. Approaching the last stage of the race, the strain is increasing, but you dig in for the final sprint towards the finish. You cross the line, exhausted but exultant.

The secret of successful visualization is realism. The more details you can cram in there—landmarks, the clothes you're wearing, other athletes, the sound of the crowd—the closer your mental race will be to the real McCoy. Come race day, all you have to do is physically follow the route your mind has gone over again and again.

Visualize it first, then execute it.

The best way to visualize a race is to view the actual course. Most competitions provide maps in advance, so practice doing the course for 1 or more of your workouts if you can, or at least drive over it in a car. Where are the hills, the sharp turns, the windy sections, the possible bottlenecks? Set the odometer and pick out some key landmarks, so you know exactly where you are and how far you have to go at every point during the race.

You've probably used elements of positive visualization in the past without even being aware of what you were doing. Negative visualization, on the other hand, is less commonly used, even by top athletes. But it's just as worthwhile. A better term for it might be "Plan B Visualization" or "Worst-Case Scenario Visualization," because you imagine all the things that could get completely screwed up during the race. Anticipating what might go wrong—and figuring out how to react and deal with each problem—can help avert potential disaster and enable you to perform at your best. What if you start out too fast? Or begin to fade halfway through? Or get a bad cramp? Many of these problems are encountered during training, so you'll know from experience to slow down or breathe differently or push on through. Perhaps even more importantly, negative visualization allows you to accept the fact that you're going to feel bad during the race. Whenever you really exert yourself physically, it's going to hurt, so make a conscious vow before the race not to give up when your body starts screaming to stop. It sounds crazy, but doing this in advance will keep you from squandering time and energy debating the matter in the heat of battle.

Start visualizing early, in Phase One if you like, and do it at least once or twice a week. It keeps you motivated, especially when you're training hard and the race seems light-years away. Practice visualization before time trials or before between-phase competitions, too, and during Phase Four, practice it several times a week. All it takes is a few minutes before, during, or after a workout or whenever you have some spare time. The one time to avoid doing visualization is right before you go to sleep. It can get the adrenaline pumping so much that sleep becomes impossible. Remember…

You can't do it if you can't imagine yourself doing it!

The 24 Hours of Race Day

Finally, the 24 hours of race day arrives. The tough part is behind you—now it's time to get out there and kick some butt. Get to the start line in fighting form by establishing a set routine for the 24 hours before the race. Find a formula that works for you, then use it before each and every race. This can take some experimenting because what works for your friends won't necessarily be a good fit for you. Use practice races to fine-tune your prerace routine. Here are a few pointers:

Don't Exercise Much the Day Before a Race

Don't make the all-too-common mistake of exercising too much the day before a race. Do a brief Active Rest Workout instead, just enough to take the edge off and keep your body loose.

What If I Can't Handle This Training Schedule?

Training for competition takes greater dedication—more time, more effort, more discipline, more sacrifices. But if getting an absolute maximum performance out of yourself is your goal, the principles outlined in the I.T. Competitive Edge Program will get you there. The program is ambitious, but it's designed so that you control the intensity level at all times, allowing you to finish each workout without completely wiping yourself out. If you're crunched for time or find you just can't handle the load physically, use common sense and scale things back. Do fewer reps for your I.T. Workouts and shorten the length of your XL Workouts and Active Rest Days. Or redirect your energies toward your I.T. or XL Workouts and cut back on the others.

Try to keep the effort level up as high as possible to get the most physiologic benefit out of I.T. Competitive Edge training. A short session is better than no session at all. It won't do as much to improve your conditioning, but it can help you maintain rhythm as your target race approaches.

Don't Do Any Strenuous Activity the Day Before a Race

Come to think of it, nix any strenuous activity the day before a race, so you don't risk getting sore or overly tired. Resting up for a race in this manner is an excellent way to avoid doing boring, heavy-duty household chores, and we recommend it highly.

Eat a Light Dinner

You don't want a heavy meal sitting in your gut at the start line. Skip the porterhouse steak the night before and eat a light dinner instead. Opt for carbohydrates over fat and protein—pasta, soups, and salads are all good bets. If you're doing a long event, such as a marathon, eat more carbs for 3 or 4 days prior to the race to increase the amount of glycogen stored in your muscles—this can keep you from "bonking" partway through the race.

Get Some Sleep

Get a good night's sleep. Or try to. But don't worry too much if you end up tossing and turning into the wee hours—many elite athletes do it, too, and still manage to compete successfully the next day. Adrenaline should carry you through.

Wake Up Early

It's never a bad idea to wake up early. Set your alarm for at least 3 hours before the race so your body has time to fully prepare for the effort that lies ahead.

Eat and/or Drink Something

Experiment well in advance of race day to find out what you can tolerate. Some people want nothing more than clear fluids before a race, such as water or sports drinks or black coffee. Others like to eat an easy-to-digest snack a couple hours ahead of time, something with about 300 calories or so. If you have a long-endurance event, it's a good idea to eat a small meal about 6 hours before the start, just to have some fuel in your system. You might want to stash some dried fruit or energy gel on your bike or in a pocket, too, just in case you run low on sugar out there on the road. No matter how long or short the race, be sure to drink up—have at least a couple of 8-ounce glasses of fluid.

Get to the Race Site Early

Getting to the race site early allows you enough time to register, if you haven't already done so, and use the bathroom. You've trained very hard for this moment, so don't let a late arrival shorten your warm-up. You need every moment.

Warm-Up

Do an easy warm-up for 5 to 15 minutes (more if the race is very short) and a handful of 10- to 30-second sprints at race pace or faster to get the heart and muscles primed for the effort ahead. Why sprint now? Think back to your I.T. Workouts and how the 1st repetition always seems so much more difficult than the next few. Basically, this is because your body would rather kick back and relax than exert itself, so it grumbles a bit as you prod it into action. These prerace sprints (with walking in between) will get that sluggish 1st rep out of the way so that you can move at a faster pace from the get-go. Time your sprints so you finish about 5 or 10 minutes before the start of the race.

Plan On Having Prerace Jitters

It's okay to feel nervous jitters before a race—in fact, it serves an important purpose. Adrenaline is a well-known performance booster and is one reason why competition can help you achieve your physical best. Move about slowly, get to the line, take a few deep breaths, and wait for the gun. You're ready.

Keep a Steady Race Pace

It's easier to maintain a steady race pace when you figure out the "splits" in advance, knowing exactly how quickly you need to complete each section of the race in order to meet your time goal. This can be tricky outside of a regulation track or pool, as you need to allow for hills, rolling terrain, or inaccurate distance markers (another good reason to check out the course beforehand). But a rough plan is still better than nothing.

Not quite sure of your abilities? Divide the race in half and hold back a bit for the first half, then push more aggressively the rest of the way to the finish.

Congratulate, Then Evaluate

When the race is over, give yourself a well-deserved pat on the back. Then take a moment to do a postmortem evaluation of your performance, relishing the good parts and learning from those less-than-stellar moments. Were you full of speed at the start but weak at the end? Focus on more XL Workouts to build endurance. Was the pace too fast? Concentrate on shorter, faster reps in your I.T. Workouts. Problems with hills? Choppy water? Wind? An upset

stomach? Make adjustments to your future workouts and prerace routine to better prepare for these situations next time.

The I.T. Competitive Edge Program for Multisport Competitions

If your ultimate goal is to perform in biathlons (two events) or triathlons (three events), the same I.T. Program training principles still apply. Be sure to realistically assess how much time and energy you can commit to this more-ambitious training. Elite athletes devote 4 to 8 hours a day to multisport training; for many of them it's a full-time job! The rest of us make do with squeezing in an hour or 2 of training time on weekdays, and maybe a bit more on weekends. With this in mind, you might consider alternating activities on weekdays and use the weekends for XL Workouts and multisport workouts (intense back-to-back workouts for two or three different sports). A multisport athlete in Phase One might train with a 14-day cycle instead of a 7-day cycle, just because the workout schedule is so much more complicated. For example, a triathlete's training week might look like the following:

Day 1: Running: I.T.
WU 10–15 min
12 x 1-min reps/2-min jog interval
CD 5–10 min

Day 2: Swimming: XL (50 min at
increased intensity)

Day 3: Cycling: I.T.
WU 10–15 min
12 x 1-min reps/2-min easy
cycling for interval
CD 5–10 min

Day 4: AR with slow running

Day 5: Swimming: I.T.
WU 10–15 min
12 x 1-min rep/2-min easy
interval
CD 5–10 min

Day 6: (weekend) Cycling: 90 min to 2
hours (moderate intensity)

Day 7: (weekend) Running: 75 min
(moderate intensity)

Day 8: Day off

Day 9: Cycling: XL (50 min, increased
intensity)

Day 10: Running: XL (50 min, increased
intensity)

Day 11: Swimming: I.T.
WU 10–15 min
12 x 1-min rep/2-min easy
interval
CD 5–10 min

Day 12: AR cycling

Day 13: Day off

Day 14: Swimming: XL (75 min, moderate
intensity)

Do 3 intense workouts in a row for each cycle, 1 for each sport, followed by an Active Rest Day.

These longer cycles work best when they stay flexible—there will be days when you can't use the pool or it's too dark outside to ride safely.

This sample schedule also doesn't include any multisport workouts, but these should be done about once every week or 2. Multisport workouts should not include 2 I.T. sessions in the same day or two XL Workouts—it's overload for training purposes and can lead to injury. Instead, do an I.T. Workout for one sport and a XL Workout for the other, and do them in the same order as in an actual competition. It's a tough day of exercise, so be sure the next day is a full day off.

Some athletes like "double days," doing 1 workout in the morning and another one later in the afternoon or evening. This is fine on occasion, if you have the time. Just make sure each workout is for a different sport, to prevent overuse injuries, and make one of the workouts no more intense than an Active Rest session. This will let you build up endurance without grinding your body down completely.

I.T. Competitive Edge Program for Long-Distance Competition

For distance events lasting more than 2 hours, such as a marathon or a century ride, endurance is the thing that will make or break you. Because of this, skip Phase Three (the Speed phase) altogether and divide your training time between Phase One and Phase Two, with 3 weeks or so set aside for Phase Four.

Use the Phase One: Long-Distance I.T. schedule to increase your XL Workouts to about 75 percent of your estimated target race time. For example, if you plan to run a marathon in 4 hours, you need to be able to run for 3 hours at a modest pace during training. To get there, gradually increase your time each week until you reach 2 hours; then, increase by no more than 5 to 15 percent every other week until you hit the 3-hour mark. On alternate weeks, continue with 2-hour sessions.

Here's an 18-week Phase One: XL Workout training cycle to prepare for a 4-hour marathon:

Week 1:	1 hour
Week 2:	1.20 hours
Week 3:	1.40 hours
Week 4:	1.60 hours
Week 5:	1.80 hours
Week 6:	2 hours
Week 7:	2 hours
Week 8:	2.20 hours
Week 9:	2 hours
Week 10:	2.40 hours
Week 11:	2 hours
Week 12:	2.60 hours
Week 13:	2 hours
Week 14:	2.80 hours
Week 15:	2 hours
Week 16:	3 hours
Week 17:	2 hours
Week 18:	3 hours

Note: Never do more than 3 hours straight training. At around 3 hours, you reach a point of diminishing returns and you just risk injury. Also, the day after each long session should be a day off to let the body adjust to the increased stress and replenish energy stores.

The other Phase One workouts remain the same.

Phase Two/XL Workouts should alternate weeks between 2 particular workouts: 1 session done for the maximum allowed time (such as the 3-hour session in the above sample); the other done for 90 minutes or half the maximum, whichever is greater. Again, give yourself a full day off after these longer sessions.

The other Phase Two workouts remain the same.

Remember to skip Phase Three!

Phase Four is the same as the regular Long-Distance I.T. Program, but you should do only one test race during this phase. Make certain it's short (less than 45 or 50 minutes) and at least 2 weeks before your target race. The final week prior to your big race should consist of nothing more than Active Rest Days to allow you to accumulate maximum fuel stores for the race ahead.

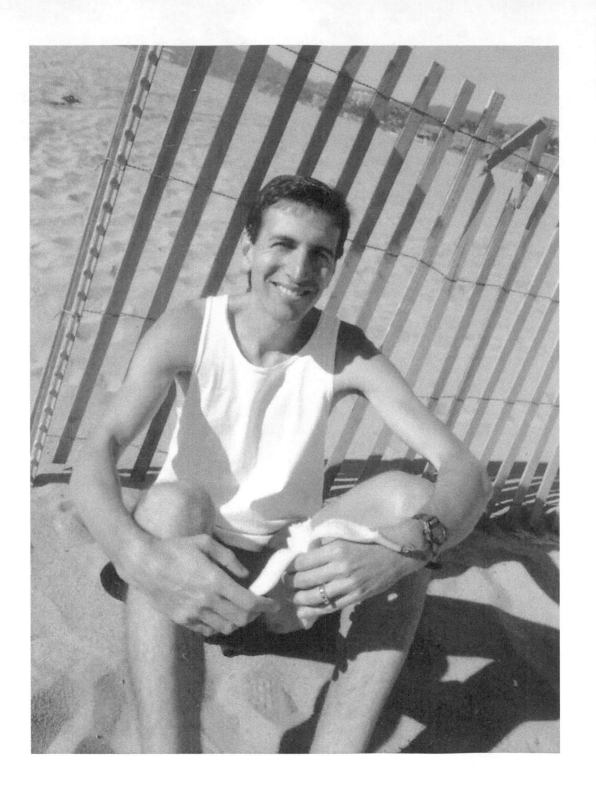

Keeping track of your workouts can help you to see progress, avoid overtraining, and find out what works best for you. Here's a sample page from one of our own workout logs so you can get an idea of how to use one. There's also a blank page for you to photocopy to make own your workout log.

Day/Date:	Monday, 8/14
Workout:	I.T.
	WU 15-min jog
	I.T. 5 x 2.5-min strides/
	2.5-min jog
	CD 10-min jog
Comments:	feel good!

Day/Date:	Tuesday, 8/15
Workout:	AR 20-min run
Comments:	tired

Day/Date:	Wednesday, 8/16
Workout:	I.T.
	WU 20-min jog
	I.T. 12 x 30-sec sprints/
	1-min jog
	CD 10 min
Comments:	still feeling a bit tired

Day/Date:	Thursday, 8/17
Workout:	day off
Comments:	

Day/Date:	Friday, 8/18
Workout:	XL 75-min run
Comments:	really hot out, but felt strong

Day/Date:	Saturday, 8/19
Workout:	AR 20-min easy swim
Comments:	left ankle sore from running, swim today

Day/Date:	Sunday, 8/20
Workout:	AR 20-min run
Comments:	ankle better today

Workout Log

(Make copies as needed)

Day/Date: _____

Workout: _____

_____

_____

_____

Comments: _____

Day/Date: _____

Workout: _____

_____

_____

_____

Comments: _____

Day/Date: _____

Workout: _____

_____

_____

_____

Comments: _____

Day/Date: _____

Workout: _____

_____

_____

_____

Comments: _____

Day/Date: _____

Workout: _____

_____

_____

_____

Comments: _____

Day/Date: _____

Workout: _____

_____

_____

_____

Comments: _____

Day/Date: _____

Workout: _____

_____

_____

_____

_____

_____

_____

(Make copies as needed)

Day/Date: _____

Workout: _____

_____

_____

_____

Comments: _____

Day/Date: _____

Workout: _____

_____

_____

_____

Comments: _____

Day/Date: _____

Workout: _____

_____

_____

_____

Comments: _____

Day/Date: _____

Workout: _____

_____

_____

_____

Comments: _____

Day/Date: _____

Workout: _____

_____

_____

_____

Comments: _____

Day/Date: _____

Workout: _____

_____

_____

_____

Comments: _____

Day/Date: _____

Workout: _____

_____

_____

_____

_____

_____

Glossary

Active Rest Days—Light exercise sessions which allow for recovery between more intense exercise.

Adenosine triphosphate (ATP)—A molecule that provides energy for cellular function. It is produced both aerobically and anaerobically and is stored within muscle and other cells.

Aerobic base—The initial training phase of the I.T. Competitive Edge Program, with an emphasis on building mitochondria, capillary density, and biomechanical efficiency.

Aerobic exercise—Exercise that allows for a continuous supply of oxygen to working muscles; usually done at a moderate intensity that can be sustained for long periods of time.

Aerobic metabolism—The primary energy source during long-distance training and racing; the efficient conversion of carbohydrates, fats, and proteins, with oxygen, to ATP.

Agonist muscle—A muscle that is mainly responsible for contraction within a particular exercise, also known as a "prime mover."

Amenorrhea—Absence of menstruation.

Anaerobic exercise—Intense exercise that overwhelms the available oxygen utilized by working muscles; usually intense physical activity that cannot be sustained for very long.

Anaerobic metabolism—The relatively inefficient conversion of carbohydrates to ATP without the assistance of oxygen.

Anaerobic threshold (AT)—The level of exercise intensity wherein more lactic acid (a waste byproduct) is produced than can be rapidly "cleared" by the body. Exercising above this threshold is difficult because lactic acid hinders energy transfer.

Antagonist muscle—A muscle that acts in opposition to an agonist muscle.

Baseline aerobic workout—The steady, low-to-moderate, comfortably paced exercise performed by most exercisers prior to the I.T. Program.

Calorie—Amount of heat required to raise the temperature of 1 cubic centimeter of water 1 degree Celsius; the basic unit used to indicate how much potential energy is contained within a given amount of food.

Carbohydrate—Nutrient supplying energy to the body, usually categorized as "simple" (e.g., sugars) and "complex" (e.g., grains, rice, beans).

Carbo-loading—A week long regimen that manipulates exercise intensity and carbohydrate consumption in order to store as much glycogen within the body as possible for use during an endurance event, such as a marathon.

Catecholamines—Naturally occurring substances such as adrenaline that the body secretes to aid in metabolism and other cell processes.

Cooldown—Gradual slowing down of activity after exercise, allowing the body to safely return to a normal state.

Cross training—Using a variety of physical activities to build strength, increase motivation, and reduce risk of injury.

Dehydration—Having less than an optimal amount of water in the body.

Duration—The length of an exercise session.

Echocardiogram—Two-dimensional ultrasound image of the heart, often used by physicians to evaluate cardiac function.

Efficiency—Ratio of energy expenditure to work output.

Electrolytes—Minerals found within the body, including sodium and potassium.

Endurance—The ability to perform repeated muscular contractions for an extended period of time.

Fartlek—A Swedish word meaning "speed play," similar to interval training except that repetitions and intervals are done in a more flexible, free-form manner.

Fat—An essential nutrient providing a source of energy to the body.

Fixed exercise machines—Gym-based workout equipment such as stair climbers, stationary bicycles, elliptical trainers, cross-country ski machines, and rowing machines.

Flexibility—Ability of the joints to move through their full range of motion.

Glucose—A simple sugar; the usual form in which carbohydrates are used as a source of energy.

Glycogen—Stored carbohydrate in muscle.

Heart rate monitor—An electronic device that provides a pulse readout during exercise.

Heart failure—Inability of the heart to manage stress.

Hydration—Taking in fluids to keep the body's water percentage at an optimal level.

Hypoglycemia—Low blood sugar.

Intensity—Degree of effort needed to accomplish a particular physical activity.

Interval (or rest)—Slower, easier period of recovery between more intense segments of a workout.

I.T. Workouts—Exercise sessions focusing on interval training, with alternating periods of intense and light activity.

Lactic acid (lactate)—A natural waste product of anaerobic energy production, causing temporary muscle fatigue and eventual muscle failure.

Mitochrondria—Cell "powerhouses" containing enzymes needed by the cell to convert food into energy.

Muscular strength—The maximum force that can be exerted by a muscle against a resistance.

Myocardial ischemia—Lack of oxygen to the heart.

Orthodics—Custom-made shoe inserts to support the foot and correct any physical imbalances (e.g., fallen arches).

Overload—Applying a greater stress to a muscle or physical system to increase strength or speed; how the body adapts in response to demands applied above a certain threshold.

Overuse injury—Injury caused by repeated activity that places too much stress on a particular body part over an extended period of time.

Periodization—A system of varying workout emphasis (endurance, stamina, speed) to attain maximum performance at a desired time.

Plateau effect—Leveling off of fitness level after an initial period of gradual improvement.

Progressive overload—Applying increased physiologic stress to muscles over a given period of time (days, months, years) to increase strength and fitness.

Protein—Essential nutrient made up of amino acids, responsible for building and repairing muscle and other tissues.

Recovery—Period of light activity (or no activity) following a race or heavy training, to allow the body to replenish energy stores and repair tissue damage.

Repetition—The high-intensity portion of an Interval Training Workout; a period of greater effort lasting from 30 seconds to about 5 minutes.

Repetition length—Duration of a repetition, as determined by either time or distance.

Repetition number—Total number of intense segments of exercise completed during an Interval Training Workout.

R.I.C.E.—Basic first aid for many minor exercise-related injuries; an acronym for Rest, Ice, Compression (with an elastic bandage to control swelling), and Elevation (putting injury above heart level to control swelling and pain).

Specificity—Training in a particular fashion in order to best perform a similar task.

Stamina—Ability to perform at a high intensity for an extended period of time.

Step up/step down method—The increased intensity/decreased intensity method of formulating a first I.T. Workout.

Strength training—Weight or resistance training.

Stress fracture—A hairline break in a bone, usually caused by overuse or improper technique.

Stress test—Walking or jogging on a treadmill under medical supervision while the heart is monitored for changes.

Stretch reflex—Extent to which a muscle can lengthen before it contracts; when a muscle stretches too far, the stretch reflex kicks in and contracts the muscle to avoid further stretching and possible injury.

Subjective assessment (or "feel")—Method of measuring intensity used most often by advanced-level athletes.

Talk test—Ability to speak during exercise; a subjective method for measuring exercise intensity.

Time trial—An individual race against the clock, performed outside of an organized competition.

Vegan—A pure vegetarian who doesn't eat any animal-derived foods.

Warm-up—Mild exercise done before stretching or a workout to prepare muscles for more intense exercise.

XL Workouts—Extra-long exercise sessions, designed to develop endurance and burn calories.

Recommended Reading

Bannister, Roger, and Frederick C. Klein. *The Four-Minute Mile.* New York: The Lyons Press, 1994.

Fixx, James F. *Complete Book of Running.* New York: Random House, 1977.

Parker, John L., Jr. *Once a Runner.* Tallahassee, FL: Cedarwinds Publishing Co., 1998.

Parker, John L., Jr. *Runners and Other Dreamers.* Tallahassee, FL: Cedarwinds Publishing Co., 1998.

Track and Field News

Runner's World

Website Sources

Cycling

bicycling.com—listings of local clubs and shops and a handy monthly events calendar

bikeleague.org—official website for the League of American Cyclists

usacycling.org—race results, event calendar, clubs, TV schedules

Medical Information

americanheart.org—the website of the American Heart Association, with a self-test for cardiovascular problems and tips on how to avoid heart disease

intelihealth.com

onhealth.com

Nutrition

athletesvillage.com—calls itself "the complete performance center for athletes," advice and instruction from elite athletes, coaches, doctors, plus a searchable database of events, clubs, and organizations

cyberdiet.com—well-presented nutrition information, over 300 recipes, low-fat cooking techniques

enutrition.com—weight management, sports nutrition, vitamins, lots of health-related news and facts

nutrition.com

PHYS.com—interactive fitness and nutrition site

Running

activeusa.com—comprehensive guide to sporting events around the USA and on-line registration for a good number of them (this site recently merged with racegate.com)

americanrunning.org—American Running Association info. on training, nutrition, injury prevention, treatment, and rehabilitation. Check out the running shoe database or the nagging injury section.

aquajogger.com—buoyancy belts for pool running, comes with a video and how-to guide: (800) 922-9544

coolrunning.com—daily national and regional running news, plus calendars, special events, forums, race listings, and results

racedates.com—Web search calendar for recreational sporting events

roadrunnersports.com—info on shoe sizing and brands, linked to its catalog

runnersworld.com

running.com—collection of links broken down into categories such as clubs, events, training, and online magazines

Swimming

fitnessswimmer.com

usa-swimming.org—info on open-water swimming

usms.org—info on open-water swimming

Triathlons

geocities.com/Colosseum/3359/tristuff.html—good tri site with links to sites specializing in triathlons, swimming, cycling, running, and fitness

multisports.com—camps, coaching, training programs, and news

trisite.com—search engine for everything dealing with triathlon, duathlon, swimming, cycling, and running

xtri.com—race results from major triathlons around the world, along with training advice, profiles, news